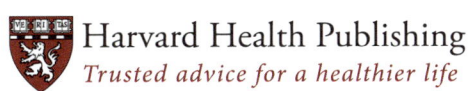 

Dear Reader,

Once seen as a fringe activity in America, yoga has gone fully mainstream, as more people have come to appreciate its wide-ranging benefits. For some, it is primarily a workout, focusing on physical postures that build strength and flexibility. For others, it is more about stress relief and meditation. Whether you start your day with a few sun salutations or adopt a more comprehensive approach, yoga can enhance your life.

The program in this report is suitable for most people who are reasonably strong and fit. If you have never tried yoga before, consider starting with our earlier Special Health Report, *An Introduction to Yoga*, which is designed to help a beginner to ease into the practice. The introductory program includes a variety of simple yoga poses and breathing exercises, along with an overview of the impressive research validating yoga's benefits.

Intermediate Yoga adopts the same general approach, but takes it several steps further. In particular, it sketches out a basic yoga routine, followed by five add-on routines with different goals in mind—enhancing flexibility, improving your balance, building strength, boosting your energy, and calming or centering yourself. You can choose whatever goal you most want to focus on at any given time. Along with the poses, each routine includes a specific breathing technique and mudra (hand position that helps focus your attention) so you can get more out of your practice. You'll also find a variety of meditations that you can do separately or with a specific practice to further your goals.

This report draws on the respective strengths of its two medical editors. One of us is a physician involved in medical education and research at the Benson-Henry Institute for Mind Body Medicine at Massachusetts General Hospital. The other is a clinical social worker and certified yoga teacher who leads yoga programs at the same hospital. Between us, we combine expertise in both the theoretical and the practical aspects of yoga—that is, a deep dive into the many mechanisms by which yoga affects the body and brain, along with the hands-on knowledge of how to structure a satisfying, safe, and fulfilling yoga practice.

We look forward to sharing this knowledge with you. So, take a deep breath, and let's get started.

Sincerely,

Darshan Mehta, M.D., M.P.H.
Medical Editor

Laura Malloy, L.I.C.S.W., C.-I.A.Y.T.
Medical Editor

Harvard Health Publishing | Harvard Medical School | 4 Blackfan Circle, 4th Floor | Boston, MA 02115

The power of yoga

Practices do not exist for thousands of years if they do not fulfill a need—and there are few practices still in use today that are older than yoga. Scholars believe that yoga has existed in India since before recorded history. Ancient soapstone seals from the Indus Valley, dating back 5,000 years, depict figures in what appear to be yogic postures. These seated figures, with their legs folded under them in apparent meditation, show no signs of fear, despite being surrounded by wild animals.

Fast-forward to 1981, when Dr. Herbert Benson, now director emeritus of the Benson-Henry Institute for Mind Body Medicine at Massachusetts General Hospital, visited a Tibetan monastery in Dharamsala, India, in the foothills of the Himalayan Mountains. With the aid of the Dalai Lama, he met practitioners of an advanced type of yoga known as g-Tummo (heat-generating) yoga. In this tradition, the monks enter deep meditative trances that demonstrate the power the mind can exert over the body. Experienced praactitioners are able to dry icy, wet sheets around their shoulders, while seated in uninsulated stone huts at frigid temperatures. Most of us would shiver uncontrollably, but the monks generated enough body heat that steam soon rose off the sheets. Dr. Benson and his team meticulously documented it in the journal *Nature*.

While this meditation is meant for only a small number of people, yoga meets a broad range of needs that permeate society today. Some types of yoga focus on providing an aerobic workout or improving posture and body mechanics. Others focus on promoting deep relaxation. All of them promote greater mindfulness.

Equally important in today's hectic world, yoga helps you reduce your stress level. As the work of Dr. Benson and many other researchers has shown, stress affects not only your mind, but also your body. According to research, up to 90% of all doctor visits can be attributed to stress-related complaints. Stress

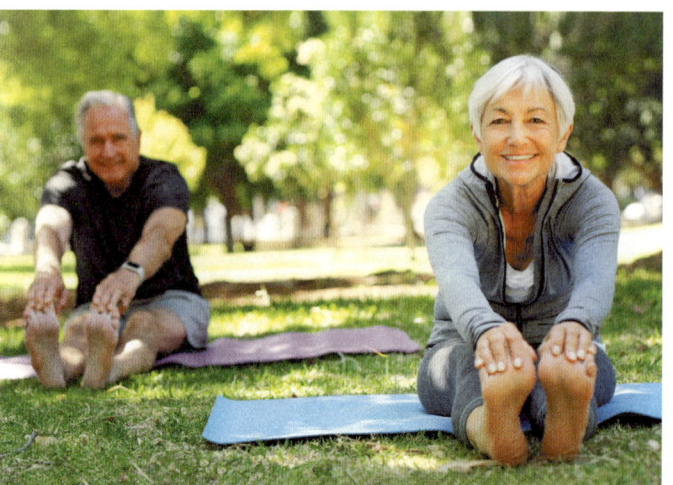

In our always plugged-in, 24/7 lives, yoga provides the respite to make you feel better—physically, mentally, and emotionally. It gives you the chance to step back and simply be present in the moment.

increases your heart rate and blood pressure, setting the stage for heart disease. It ratchets up levels of glucose (sugar) in your bloodstream, making diabetes management more difficult. It may even contribute to some forms of cancer. Yoga may help all of these.

In sum, in our always-plugged-in, 24/7 lives, yoga provides the respite to make you feel better—physically, mentally, and emotionally. It is arguably the one tool we have that simultaneously improves strength, balance, and flexibility, while helping to dial back negative self-talk and ruminations. Countering the daily pressures and demands of modern life, yoga gives you an opportunity to step back and simply be present in the moment.

In the next chapter, we'll explore some of the research into yoga's impressive effects on health and well-being. For the moment, suffice it to say that an important indicator of yoga's success appears to be in the numbers—not just in points off of blood pressure readings or cholesterol counts, but in health care bills. According to a Harvard study published in the journal *PLOS One*, when researchers compared medical costs for 4,400 people before and after they underwent relaxation training, which included yoga and meditation, they found that people used 43% fewer medical services and reaped estimated savings ranging from $640 to $25,500 per person each year.

In this report, we will help you develop your yoga practice, whether you just want a good workout or you're looking for more targeted benefits. We provide six routines that include many of the classic yoga postures you'll encounter in most yoga classes. But we tailor the workouts to help you achieve specific goals. In the morning, you may want to try the Energizing Practice (page 41), while later on, after a tough workday, you might prefer the Calming Practice (page 44). If you're feeling stiff or you need to improve the range of motion in certain joints, the Flexibility Practice (page 28) may be just the ticket. The Strengthening Practice (page 38) helps build your muscles, which can be especially useful as you naturally start to lose muscle mass with the passage of time. Or you might need to work on your balance—a skill that tends to diminish with age—by working on the Balance Practice (page 33). We also include a variety of breathing exercises that can calm, energize, or center you, along with a variety of mudras—that is, hand positions used during breathing exercises or meditation to help bring your mind into focus.

First, however, we'd like to provide some basic information about what yoga is—and is not.

What is yoga?

Translated literally, the Sanskrit term for yoga (*yuj*) means to yoke, unite, or join—specifically, to unite the body, mind, and spirit. But how do you do that? Yoga covers a broad range of practices that mean many things to many people.

Most Americans think of yoga as a workout, focusing primarily on the physical practice that is portrayed in media images. While yoga can certainly provide a good workout, it is more than just physical exercise. Yoga is a mind-body practice that has become one of the top complementary health approaches in this country, according to the National Institutes of Health. Its goals are to cultivate balance, calm, harmony, and awareness—and, in classic yoga traditions, to strive for the attainment of selflessness and spiritual enlightenment. In one survey, about 24% of the respondents listed "spiritual development" as a reason for doing yoga.

As you will see in this report, there are various components to a complete yoga practice—including postures, breathing practices, and meditation—and there are many different forms of yoga, from slow-paced to vigorous. But at the heart of it, yoga is about personal transformation. For some people, that transformation involves becoming more fit and developing a greater sense of well-being. For others, the transformation involves an entire lifestyle—including healthy behaviors (such as eating a vegetarian diet, drinking little or no alcohol, and abstaining from tobacco), practicing mindfulness, and cultivating a moral, nonviolent, and nonharming approach to others.

While yoga has traditionally been associated with Hinduism and Buddhism, it is compatible with all the world's major religions. In fact, the regular practice of yoga—which is built on the promotion of kindness and compassion toward yourself and others—may enable you to better fulfill the tenets of your own religious faith, whatever that may be.

For all these reasons, it's not surprising to learn that yoga differs from a traditional workout in some important ways. For most workouts, the goal is to do more and work harder. Yoga is more about undoing—relaxing, releasing, and letting go. You don't have to break a sweat or compete with other people. In fact, when you stop doing that, you're able to go deeper into your practice and reap more benefits. Instead of letting your mind wander or watching a TV monitor while you're on the treadmill at the gym, you will engage more fully in what you are doing in the present moment. When you're focusing in this manner, you are more likely to experience peace, calmness, and joy. Many people take up yoga as a workout, but they stick with it because it makes them happier.

The major components of yoga

Part of the reason yoga has such broad-ranging benefits is that it has not just one component, but many. Some 2,000 years ago, an Indian sage named Patanjali codified yoga, collecting existing practices into the classic text *The Yoga Sutras*. Patanjali described a holistic system encompassing eight essential paths, or "limbs," of yoga. The practices in these various limbs include both physical and mental exercises. The ones you are most likely to encounter in yoga classes today—the same ones we focus on in this report—are yoga postures, breathing exercises, and meditation. But Patanjali also included exercises aimed at fostering an ethical life (characterized by truthfulness, moderation, nonviolence, generosity, and compassion), exercising self-discipline, learning to accept oneself and others, and increasing one's powers of concentration and detachment from the world. These are an important part of a yogic lifestyle.

The more limbs you practice, the better. But even if you focus only on postures, breathing practices, and meditation, you will reap considerable benefits. Among these three, some styles of yoga and some instructors put a greater emphasis on one component or another. For example, a gym class may emphasize the physical postures. In this report, we include all three, because each of them acts in a different way, with complementary effects.

Postures (asanas)

These are the physical positions such as warrior, downward-facing dog, and tree pose that most people associate with a yoga practice. There are standing poses, seated postures, supine and prone positions, forward folds, back bends, balance poses, hip openers, twists, and inversions. Some of the postures and movements are large and overt, while others are small and subtle—and some are even purely internal or imagined motion. In different types of yoga, asanas are executed in a variety of ways. Some approaches involve holding postures for several minutes. Others require you to move rapidly from one pose to another. No matter how the postures are done, proper alignment is key to avoiding injuries and maximizing results.

The benefits from postures and movement include improved range of motion, strength, endurance, flexibility, and balance. In addition, they promote body awareness, both of internal sensations and, externally, of your body's orientation in the space around it.

Breathing practices (pranayama)

In many modern yoga practices, the breath is linked to movement as you flow from one posture to the next. But yoga also includes a number of breathing techniques that may be practiced on their own without movement—ranging from very slow and deep breathing to rapid, shallower breaths. In meditation, the breath is often a focal point to help you develop awareness. The type of breathing you do usually depends upon the style of yoga you practice and the desired effect. Some breathing techniques can even be performed throughout the day—for example, while you're driving or when you're at work—as a way to calm down and release tension.

Your breath can have a direct physiological effect on your body. Slow, rhythmic breathing promotes a balanced, relaxed state. Your heart rate slows, and hormones that promote feelings of calm and social bonding increase. The opposite happens with fast, superficial patterns of breathing. Rapid, shallow breaths activate the part of the nervous system that governs the fight-or-flight response. As a result, heart rate increases, and stress hormones are released, at least over the short term.

The most common breathing patterns in yoga are slow and rhythmic and are generally safe for beginners. Before you try more intense or rapid breathing practices (such as the breath of fire, or *kapalabhati*), check with your doctor if you have cardiac or respiratory problems, high blood pressure, diabetes, dizziness, or digestive issues such as ulcers or colitis. It is also best to practice vigorous breathing techniques under the instruction of a qualified yoga teacher.

Meditation (dhyana)

Traditionally, the purpose of the preceding components of yoga—postures and breathing—was to prepare a person for meditation. Postures and breathing can help rid you of external distractions and tension in your body, thus enabling better internal focus.

Many experts consider meditation to be the most important component of yoga, especially in our culture, because it provides a much-needed breather for our overworked, overstimulated brains. Imaging stud-

Continued on page 6

More meditations to try

The yoga practices in this report feature a basic breathing meditation. But there are many types of meditation that you can use by themselves or with any of the routines in this report.

Guided imagery

If you are a visually oriented person, using mental images may make meditation easier. In a yoga session, an instructor may talk you through a series of images. But you can also do this on your own.

Sit or lie comfortably. Clear your mind while taking deep, even breaths for several minutes. Then conjure up an image of a safe or special haven (perhaps a lake cabin, a beach house, your grandmother's kitchen, or a garden) and imagine yourself there. Allow all of your senses to be present. What do you smell—pine needles, rain steaming off hot pavement, vanilla in the kitchen? What do you hear and see? Are clouds or birds passing by? Bask in the surrounding colors. Concentrate on sensory pleasures: a cool breeze on your cheek, gravel crunching underfoot, or the scent of flowering trees. When intrusive thoughts pop into your head, simply observe them without reacting to them. Then return to your focus. Practice for 10 to 20 minutes.

Loving-kindness meditation

The loving-kindness meditation, also called metta, encourages compassion and may actually help keep you younger longer by increasing levels of the enzyme telomerase (see "Why yoga has so many benefits," page 10).

Sit in a position that is comfortable for you—perhaps cross-legged on the floor, or in a chair with your spine straight and feet flat on the floor. Your hands can rest on your knees or lie relaxed in your lap. Relax your whole body and close your eyes. Then imagine what you wish for your life and come up with three or four phrases that describe your desires—for example, "May I be healthy. May I be happy. May I be loved." As you breathe deeply, repeat these phrases to yourself several times, sending love and warmth to yourself.

Next, direct the phrases toward someone you feel thankful for or who has helped you, such as a mentor: "May you be healthy. May you be happy. May you be loved."

Continue this practice, visualizing and directing the phrases toward the following people in turn:

- a dear friend
- an acquaintance you feel neutral about—someone you neither like nor dislike
- someone you dislike or with whom you are having a difficult time
- everyone in the world.

Yoga nidra

Nidra is the Sanskrit word for "sleep." Although the term dates back through the ages, modern research has shown that it can indeed help facilitate sleep.

This practice combines meditation, breath awareness, and guided imagery to achieve a deep state of relaxation, taking you all the way to a near-sleep-like state. You can practice it at any time of the day, but if you want to get a better night's sleep, try it in bed at night. It is easiest to get started by listening to someone direct you through the practice. Search online to find free recordings.

Kirtan kriya meditation

The kirtan kriya meditation—also called "sa-ta-na-ma" meditation—comes from the Kundalini yoga tradition (see "Selecting a type of yoga," page 47). It involves finger movements as well as a spoken mantra and is said to be good for mental clarity. In studies of people with mild cognitive impairment—and their highly stressed caregivers—it helped reduce depression and anxiety and improve sleep.

Sit in a position that is comfortable for you, with your hands resting in your lap and the index finger and thumb of each hand touching at the fingertips, in a classic hand position called the wisdom mudra, or *gyan mudra* (see "Wisdom and consciousness mudras," page 27). Close your eyes, and take a few deep breaths.

As you recite the mantra sa-ta-na-ma out loud, you will press different fingers together:

- On "sa," press the thumb and index finger of each hand together.
- On "ta," press the thumb and middle finger together.
- On "na," press the thumb and ring finger together.
- On "ma," press the thumb and little finger together.

Repeat this nine more times, continuing to recite the syllables of the mantra aloud.

Repeat 10 more times, saying the syllables in a whisper.

Repeat the cycle silently. Finish with a few deep breaths before opening your eyes.

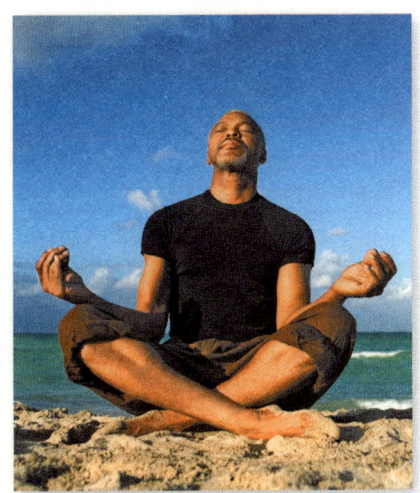

Continued from page 4

ies show that during meditation, people can engage the frontal lobe connections that directly affect the limbic system, the part of the brain that controls emotions. The resulting changes in brain activity—and, over the long term, even in brain structure—enable you to better manage stress and to handle negative emotions like fear, anger, depression, and anxiety in more positive ways.

There are many different types of meditation, but all involve the relaxed and persistent focus of attention in a nonanalytical way. A common way to meditate is to focus on a single target such as a mantra (a repeated word or phrase), your breath, or a candle. Another common form is called mindfulness meditation, in which awareness is centered on the flow of sensation or the flow of thought itself. It is common, especially when you are just learning to meditate, for your mind to wander and for thoughts like "I need to pay the electric bill" to pop into your head. That's okay; everyone who meditates has episodes of the mind wandering or thoughts intruding. Simply acknowledge the errant thought and bring your focus back to your target without being judgmental or trying to analyze it.

Some instructors use guided meditations, such as loving-kindness meditation (see page 5), in which they talk you through a mental exercise of sending compassion and kindness to others. Or they may use guided imagery (see page 5), describing a location such as a beach and sensations such as the warmth of the sun for you to imagine as you meditate.

If meditation is part of a yoga session, it is generally done at the end. However, you can also practice meditation throughout a session by focusing your attention on either the movements you are doing or on your breath. You can meditate while sitting, lying, standing, or even moving, once you are experienced. Ultimately, the goal is to carry over this practice into daily living, so that you go about your day more mindfully. While eating dinner, for example, you'll pay attention to the tastes and textures of your food, thus deriving deeper satisfaction from them, rather than working or surfing the Internet while you eat and largely ignoring the food you're consuming.

The wisdom of combining components

Each of these three practices—postures, breathing exercises, and meditation—affects you in a different way. Combined, they can be quite powerful.

Physical fitness. Your balance, flexibility, strength, coordination, and breathing capacity improve. These changes result primarily from the physical postures and breathing techniques.

Better management of emotions and stress. Volatile emotions become more stable. You handle stress better. You're more resilient when faced with problems. Your self-efficacy—that is, your belief in your ability to function effectively—increases. Meditation is the key component that improves self-regulation of thought processes, which underlies stress reduction and the ability to regulate your emotions. However, breathing practices and other components also contribute.

Mind-body awareness or mindfulness. As you tune in to the subtle cues of your body, you become more aware of the consequences of your behaviors. For example, when you eat a lot of junk food, you notice that your body doesn't feel good. By contrast, when you do something positive like exercise, you're more aware of the physical and mental benefits that flow from it. As a result, you start to gravitate toward positive behaviors and away from negative ones. Meditation is the primary component that promotes mind-body awareness.

Spirituality. This deeper experience comes with more practice and creates a sense of unity, oneness, peace, harmony, flow, or even expanded consciousness. You gain more meaning and purpose in your life. Increased spirituality can be transformative, influencing your values, your relationships, your goals, and the way you live your life.

The health benefits of yoga

For too long, Western medicine regarded the mind and body as separate entities with no influence on each other. In recent years, however, research has made it abundantly clear that the two are inextricably linked. The body has powerful effects on the mind, and vice versa. A practice like yoga, which directly targets both, is considered to be a form of mind-body exercise—and one of the most powerful. Although the scientific study of its benefits is relatively new, researchers are rapidly developing a body of evidence documenting the benefits of yoga for both physical and mental health, not to mention overall well-being.

On a practical level, this is reflected in the number of times yoga is now being mentioned in electronic medical records. According to a 2019 study in the *Journal of the American Board of Family Medicine*, notations on the therapeutic use of yoga increased more than 10-fold from 2006 to 2016 at a large academic medical center in Pennsylvania. Doctors recommended yoga for conditions as diverse as anxiety, high cholesterol, fatigue, muscle pain, and Parkinson's disease.

Whether your goal is to bring down your blood pressure, improve your strength and flexibility, boost your mood, or just get some exercise, yoga can help. This chapter provides a brief overview of some of the benefits.

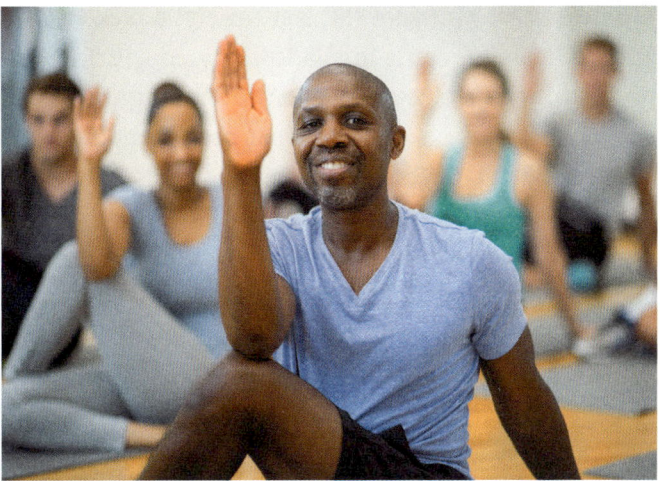

Yoga helps improve your flexibility, balance, strength, coordination, and breathing capacity. It can also improve your mental state and overall well-being.

Increased well-being

If you wanted to improve your well-being, what are some of the things you might wish for? Better sleep, perhaps? More energy? Would you like to trim off five pounds? How about being more content with yourself and more resilient in the face of challenges that inevitably come your way? Even at this early stage of research, scientists have indications that yoga can help with all of these and more. What makes these findings so exciting is that they suggest that a regular yoga practice can improve multiple areas of your life at once, creating positive feedback loops that can further promote health. For example, yoga can help improve your sleep, which in turn gives you more energy and focus during your day. When you feel better physically and mentally, you have the energy to adopt better habits, including a healthier diet and more physical activity. More exercise in turn can improve your sleep, and so the cycle continues.

Less stress, greater resilience

Stress abounds in our lives. Much of the time, there's little you can do to change the outside world—you can't wish away a traffic jam or make an airline un-cancel a flight. What you *can* change is how you perceive stressful situations and how resilient you are—that is, how able you are to adapt to and recover from stress.

Yoga helps you learn to react less emotionally when stressful situations inevitably arise. Research has shown that a single 90-minute yoga session can lower levels of cortisol, a stress hormone that puts your body into an excited state as opposed to a relaxed one. While a certain amount of cortisol is necessary and even helpful under the right circumstances, too much cortisol on a sustained basis wreaks havoc on your body, which is why yoga's stress-reduction benefits are so powerful (see "Why yoga has so many benefits," page 10).

When it comes to countering stress, one of the important tools yoga provides is a variety of breathing practices. Think of the last time you were upset, and your breath came in shallow, jagged spurts. Simply slowing and deepening your breathing calms the autonomic nervous system—that part of the nervous system that operates largely beyond your conscious control, governing bodily functions like heart rate and digestion. Deep breathing dials back cortisol levels and helps put you into a calmer state. As you strive to unite the mind, body, and spirit in a healthy whole, breath is key, forging a sturdy central link among the three.

Better sleep

How do you feel when you wake up in the morning—refreshed and ready to go, or groggy and grumpy? As many as one in three Americans sleeps less than six hours a night. Insufficient sleep can make you too tired to work efficiently, to exercise, or to eat healthfully. Over time, sleep deprivation increases the risks for a number of chronic health problems, including heart disease, stroke, and diabetes. But emerging research shows that yoga may help you fall asleep faster, sleep longer, and sleep more soundly—without the negative side effects of medication.

Yoga facilitates sleep by reducing stress, anxiety, and arousal—all known causes of poor sleep. A national survey reported that over 55% of people who did yoga said that it helped them get better sleep. According to the National Sleep Foundation, pregnant women who start a mindful yoga practice in their second trimester sleep better and wake up less through the night, and cancer patients sleep better despite the disruptive effects of chemotherapy.

Better balance, flexibility, and body awareness

It's easy to see why yoga promotes flexibility. As you move more deeply into poses, muscle fibers and connective tissues gradually relax, allowing greater range of motion. Pictures of longtime yogis in seemingly impossible postures demonstrate just how much flexibility you can develop over time. But even if you increase your flexibility just a little, it can help you accomplish everyday tasks with greater ease and avoid certain types of injuries.

Your sense of balance also improves with a regular yoga practice. Balance is a more complicated phenomenon than you might imagine. It requires the coordination of multiple bodily systems—the musculoskeletal system (muscles, tendons, and bones), of course, but also the central nervous system, the vestibular system in the inner ear, the visual processing system in the brain, and proprioceptors (position-sensing parts of nerves). As you hold a variety of postures, you hone all these systems, and your proprioception (the sense of where your body is in space) becomes more keen.

Greater awareness of your body can have many payoffs over time. You may find that your posture improves, allowing you to take deeper breaths. Better posture also leads to more efficient body mechanics. This can help you to move with more ease and may even reduce your risk of falling or help you recover if you stumble.

Weight loss

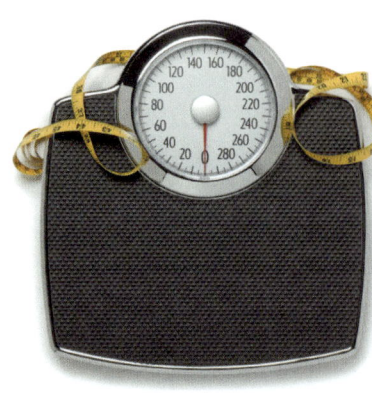

If you're trying to lose weight, you may think that activities like boot camp or Zumba would be most likely to help you shed pounds. While it's unlikely you'll burn as many calories, research suggests that yoga works, but in different ways. For one thing, it promotes better sleep, which in turn improves the balance of hormones in your body that govern hunger and satiety. When you're sleep-deprived, you tend to crave more sugary, high-calorie food. When you sleep more soundly, a better hormonal balance can help dial back those cravings.

Furthermore, as you cultivate a sense of mindfulness or awareness, you may begin eating more mindfully, which can result in greater satisfaction from your meals, so you can be content with less. And because you notice when you are full (or approaching full—the traditional Indian health system of Ayurveda advocates stopping at 75%), you stop eating before you have overindulged. Furthermore, if you're less stressed, it stands to reason that you'll be less likely to turn to chips or ice cream to help you calm down. You'll also release less of the stress hormone cortisol, which has been implicated in contributing to abdominal fat.

Greater compassion, gratitude, and happiness

Researchers in the field of positive psychology have identified the leading factors that contribute to a person's sense of happiness, fulfillment, and general contentedness. A number of these factors—gratitude, compassion, savoring the moment, finding meaning in life, and flow—are things that can be enhanced with yoga and the mindfulness it can inspire.

Simply being present in the moment—a practice engendered by yoga—can lead to increased happiness by helping you to savor pleasure, consciously enjoying an experience as it unfolds. Most people are primed to experience pleasure in special moments, such as a wedding day or a vacation. Everyday pleasures, on the other hand, can slip by without much notice unless you learn to savor them. If you're walking the dog on a beautiful path but worrying about your day's to-do list, you're missing the moment.

Similarly, research has shown that yoga can increase your sense of gratitude—thankful appreciation for what you receive, whether tangible or intangible, large or small. With gratitude, you acknowledge the goodness in your life. Gratitude helps you relish positive experiences, build stronger relationships, and be more resilient in the face of adversity. In positive psychology, it consistently correlates with greater happiness and contentedness. According to a study in the *Journal of Bodywork and Movement Therapies*, the longer you practice yoga, the greater your feelings of gratitude will be for everything you have and the greater your sense of meaning in life.

Yoga also puts emphasis on living in accordance with ethical principles. Doing so not only puts you in a better frame of mind, but also reduces the cognitive dissonance that comes from behaving in ways that you know deep down are wrong. As a result, you live in greater harmony with the world.

Better physical health

Some of the previous entries touched on aspects of physical health, which is not surprising given the mind-body connection we mentioned earlier. These benefits can add up in ways that help you manage some very specific diseases. Heart disease and diabetes are two of the most important, but there are others. Preliminary research also shows that yoga may help with neck pain, multiple sclerosis, headaches, Parkinson's disease, menopause, and fibromyalgia. There is also significant research on its benefits for cancer patients and survivors, including fewer treatment side effects, improved mood, and better quality of life.

Better heart health

For nearly a century, diseases of the heart have been the No. 1 cause of death in America, claiming more lives each year than all forms of cancer combined. Yoga benefits the heart and the entire circulatory system in many ways at once.

Reduced blood pressure. Most people would never realize they had high blood pressure if their doctors didn't tell them, since the ailment has no symptoms or warning signs. But high blood pressure (hypertension) is known as "the silent killer" for good reason. It sets you up for heart attacks, strokes, and ultimately heart failure.

One 2019 analysis, published in *Mayo Clinic Proceedings*, examined 49 controlled studies and found that participants who engaged in an hourlong yoga session roughly five times a week for 13 weeks saw moderate reductions in both systolic and diastolic blood pressure (the top and bottom numbers in a blood pressure reading). Yoga practitioners had average reductions of 6 points of systolic pressure and 3 points of diastolic pressure, while people who did not do yoga saw no such improvements. When postures were combined with breathing techniques and meditation, the reductions roughly doubled—to 11 points systolic and 6 points diastolic. The authors concluded that yoga is a viable lifestyle therapy for treating high blood pressure.

Other measures of heart health. A review of randomized controlled trials, published in the *European Journal of Preventive Cardiology*, found that yoga

Continued on page 11

Why yoga has so many benefits

Researchers still have a long way to go before they will fully understand just why yoga has such a broad range of physical and mental benefits. Here's what's clear at this point.

It tamps down stress. Stress that you encounter on a daily basis doesn't just grind you down mentally. It also affects your physical health. Stress causes your body and brain to invoke the so-called fight-or-flight response—the classic stress response, which primes your body to deal with an immediate short-term threat in which you must fight an enemy or flee to safety. In the stress response, a flood of stress hormones increases your heart rate in order to pump more blood to muscles; it also releases more glucose into the bloodstream to fuel those muscles, ratchets up inflammation to deal with any potential wounds, and diverts the body's resources away from functions like digestion, which are not needed for escaping the threat.

Its opposite, the relaxation response—sometimes referred as the rest-and-digest response—calms your body. It conserves and restores energy, slowing your heart rate and lowering your blood pressure. It's responsible for maintaining functions such as digestion at the status quo. It's active when you're relaxed—and it's enhanced by yoga. Many of the benefits of yoga are the result of stress reduction and its related effects on the body.

It reduces inflammation. As noted above, reducing stress can also dial back inflammation, which has been a major focus of research in recent years, as evidence increasingly shows its potential long-term harms. To be sure, short-term inflammation is essential for survival. If you cut yourself, it aids in fighting bacteria and healing the wound. But over the long term, low-grade chronic inflammation is associated with a range of harmful effects, including the development of heart disease, diabetes, and cancer. A 2019 review of 15 yoga studies found that yoga reduced markers of inflammation.

It tones the vagus nerve. The vagus nerve winds from your brainstem down through your neck and the trunk of your body. One of 10 cranial nerves, it has been referred to as the body's "air traffic controller" because it helps regulate all major bodily functions, including your breathing, heart rate, and digestion. The two-way message traffic it coordinates between the brain and the body has an important impact on your mood and emotional regulation.

The vagus nerve is a key component of your parasympathetic nervous system (the part that governs the relaxation response). Greater vagal tone—that is, greater activity of the vagus nerve—means that your body can shift more easily from the stress response to the relaxation response. Vagal tone can't be measured directly. Instead, other biological processes—such as your heart rate during inhalations and exhalations—serve as indicators of vagal tone. When vagal tone is high, your heart is beating properly, your digestion is good, your moods are stable, and you're able to handle challenges or stress and recover from it quickly, making you more resilient in the face of stress.

If you have low vagal tone, you're more likely to have a high heart rate, sluggish digestion, a sense of being drained, and trouble controlling your moods and emotions. Conditions such as depression, chronic pain, and post-traumatic stress disorder are associated with low vagal tone. Yoga appears to increase vagal tone, providing a possible explanation for why these conditions respond well to yoga.

It increases immunity. By fighting stress and inflammation, yoga appears to improve your body's natural defenses as well. Among other things, it raises levels of your body's own antioxidants. Antioxidants neutralize free radicals (byproducts of the body's energy production or of exposure to air pollution and ultraviolet rays), which cause oxidative stress that can damage DNA, cells, and tissues and lead to disease. In a review of 11 studies, published in the *Journal of Complementary and Integrative Medicine*, yoga improved antioxidant levels and reduced oxidative stress in healthy people as well as those with diabetes, prediabetes, high blood pressure, and kidney disease.

It regulates gene expression. A review of 18 studies found that mind-body practices such as yoga and meditation generally reduce the expression (activity) of genes linked to chronic low-grade inflammation—the kind of inflammation that contributes to many serious ailments, such as heart disease. In addition to tamping down the activity of a number of disease-promoting genes, mind-body practices appear to boost that of numerous *health*-promoting genes. One of the studies included in the review showed that a simple meditation practice could upregulate (activate) certain beneficial genes in both longtime practitioners and novices. While meditation had greater and more consistent effects on the genes of the experienced practitioners, the novices also saw positive changes after eight weeks of a daily practice, resulting in the enhanced expression of genes associated with energy metabolism, mitochondrial function, insulin secretion, and telomere maintenance (all good things).

It protects your genes. It may sound improbable, but research suggests that yoga could also help keep you young—or at least, keep your cells from aging quite as fast. The key is the length of your telomeres; these are repetitive stretches of DNA at the ends of chromosomes, which serve as protective caps, much like the plastic tips on the ends of shoelaces. Shorter telomeres are associated with disease and aging, and chronic stress is a culprit in this process. But dialing back stress through yoga may help protect your telomeres. Researchers found that doing a daily 12-minute yoga meditation increased the activity of telomerase (the enzyme that helps maintain and even rebuild telomeres) by 43%. This pilot study was published in the *International Journal of Geriatric Psychiatry*.

Continued from page 9

can have a beneficial impact on additional risk factors for heart disease, including cholesterol levels, triglycerides, heart rate, and excess body weight. When compared with people who didn't do yoga or other exercise, participants averaged the following improvements after practicing yoga for an average of 12 weeks:
- 5-pound weight loss
- 18-point drop in total cholesterol
- 12-point drop in LDL (bad) cholesterol
- 3-point gain in HDL (good) cholesterol
- 6-point drop in triglycerides
- 5-point drop in systolic blood pressure
- 5-point drop in diastolic blood pressure
- 5-point drop in heart rate.

Fewer heart rhythm disturbances. Atrial fibrillation—a common disorder in which the heart beats irregularly and rapidly—affects more than 35 million people worldwide and increases the risk of stroke and death. When 538 people with the condition practiced yoga every other day for 30 minutes a session, they reported nearly 50% fewer episodes of atrial fibrillation compared with when they didn't do yoga, according to a study presented in 2020 at the European Society of Cardiology Congress.

Improved diabetes management

Learning that you have diabetes can be distressing, even traumatic. But a regular yoga practice can play a role in diabetes management.

Research has found that people who do yoga have significant reductions in their levels of blood glucose and HbA1c (a marker reflecting your average blood sugar level over the preceding two to three months). Yoga may even reduce the need for diabetes medications. In one study, people who practiced yoga for three months were able to decrease their diabetes drugs by 26% to 40%. (But don't change any of your medications without consulting with your doctor first.) It's not completely clear how yoga does this, but it may have to do with weight loss. When you lose weight, your insulin sensitivity improves, bringing down blood sugar.

Yoga's role in reducing risk factors for heart disease is also important for people with diabetes, who are at increased risk of heart disease.

Pain relief

Research suggests that yoga has benefits for people with many types of chronic pain, most notably low back pain and arthritis, but some studies have shown it can also help in easing neck pain, migraines, and even fibromyalgia. For pain relief, you should probably avoid the more strenuous forms of yoga (see "Selecting a type of yoga," page 47). Be aware that yoga postures can be modified to accommodate your strength and medical issues.

Back pain relief. Back pain is one of the most common health problems, affecting four out of five Americans at some point. Yoga helps alleviate back pain by increasing flexibility and muscle strength. Relaxation, stress reduction, and better body awareness may also play a role. A 2020 review of 23 yoga trials, published in the journal *Preventive Medicine*, found that yoga decreased pain, reduced depression and anxiety associated with back pain, and improved function. A 2017 study found that it was as effective as physical therapy for improving function and pain.

Less arthritis pain. The pain and stiffness of osteoarthritis can hamper physical activity. Yoga offers a gentle form of exercise that helps improve range of motion and strengthen the muscles around painful joints. In a study in *Current Rheumatology Reports*, eight to 12 weeks of yoga, about an hour a week, decreased pain and stiffness and improved function.

People with rheumatoid arthritis, an autoimmune disorder, may also benefit. According to research, those who do yoga report better physical health, walking ability, pain levels, energy, and mood; have significantly fewer swollen and tender joints; and are more likely to be able to work full-time than those who don't practice yoga.

Asthma relief

Asthma is a major public health problem in the Untied States, and it's been increasing in all age, sex, and racial groups. In this chronic condition, the airways constrict, causing wheezing, chest tightness, coughing, and shortness of breath. In many people, asthma is triggered by exposure to allergens. But the fear of asthma attacks can contribute to anxiety that further tightens the airways. So, it makes sense that yoga, with its breathing exercises and meditation, may help people with asthma manage these symptoms. Improvements in breathing may reduce physiological triggers of asthma attacks. Both techniques may help by reducing stress, which can exacerbate symptoms. Even postures may help by expanding the chest. More research is needed, but preliminary findings suggest that yoga may help reduce symptoms and improve quality of life for people with asthma.

Better mental health

With its emphasis on breathing practices and meditation—both of which help calm and center the mind—it's hardly surprising that yoga also brings mental benefits, such as reduced anxiety and depression. What may be more surprising is that it actually makes your brain work better.

A sharper brain

When you lift weights, your muscles get stronger and bigger. When you do yoga, your brain cells develop new connections, and changes occur in brain structure as well as function, resulting in improved cognitive skills, such as learning and memory. Yoga strengthens parts of the brain that play a key role in memory, attention, awareness, thought, and language. Think of it as weight lifting for the brain.

Structural brain changes. The use of MRI scans and other brain imaging technology has allowed scientists to observe these changes. In studies, people who did yoga had a thicker cerebral cortex (the area of the brain responsible for information processing) and hippocampus (the area of the brain involved in learning and memory) compared with nonpractitioners. These areas of the brain typically shrink as you age, but the older yoga practitioners showed less shrinkage than those who did no yoga. This suggests that yoga may counteract age-related declines in memory and other cognitive skills, even in people with cognitive decline or dementia.

Improved function. Research also shows that yoga and meditation improve executive functions, such as reasoning, decision making, memory, learning, reaction time, and accuracy on tests of mental acuity.

Improved mood

All exercise boosts mood. It burns off stress hormones, increases the production of feel-good chemicals known as endorphins, and brings more oxygenated blood to your brain. But yoga may have added benefits. One of the ways yoga appears to affect mood is by elevating levels of a brain chemical called gamma-aminobutyric acid (GABA), which is associated with better mood and decreased anxiety.

Compared with nonpractitioners, people who engage in yoga regularly also have more activity in the left prefrontal cortex of the brain. This is considered the "happy side" of the brain, and people with more activity in this area are generally more joyful. Meditation also reduces activity in the limbic system—the part of the brain dedicated to emotions. As your emotional reactivity diminishes, you have a more tempered response when faced with stressful situations.

Less depression and anxiety. Drugs and talk therapy have traditionally been the go-to remedies for depression and anxiety. But complementary approaches such as yoga are becoming more accepted, and yoga stacks up well when compared with other complementary therapies.

A review of 15 studies, published in the journal *Aging and Mental Health*, looked at the effect of a variety of relaxation techniques on depression and anxiety in older adults. In addition to yoga, interventions included massage therapy, progressive muscle relaxation, stress management, and listening to music. While all the techniques provided some benefit, yoga and music were the most effective for both depression and anxiety. And yoga appeared to provide the longest-lasting effect.

Help for PTSD. A number of small studies have found that yoga can help with post-traumatic stress disorder (PTSD). It is not used by itself, but as an add-on treatment to help reduce intrusive memories and emotional arousal and to produce calmer, steadier breathing. Deep, slow breathing is associated with calmer states, because it helps activate the parasympathetic nervous system (see "Why yoga has so many benefits," page 10).

A great deal more research is needed. But the evidence to date is already strong enough to conclude that yoga can provide comprehensive benefits. ♥

Before you start: Safety first

Even though you may have been practicing yoga for some time, now is not the time to get complacent about safety. While yoga is as safe as or safer than most forms of exercise, it's still wise to know your limits, especially as you take your practice to the next level and try more challenging routines. If you have any of the medical conditions listed in this chapter, you should consult with your doctor before starting the program. In the unlikely event that you should experience an emergency (see "Red flags that warrant a call to 911," below right), contact a doctor immediately.

In later chapters, we provide general tips on avoiding injuries during your yoga practice (see "Tips for a better, safer practice," page 16; "Avoiding injuries in class," page 52; and "Dangerous poses," page 52).

When to get a doctor's approval

The most common risk factor for injuries in yoga is having a significant medical condition. Consult your doctor before trying yoga or taking your practice to the next level if you have (or had) any of the following:

- heart disease or high blood pressure
- diabetes
- osteoporosis
- respiratory problems
- glaucoma
- balance problems
- recent surgery
- musculoskeletal problems such as back or joint problems, including a herniated disc
- stroke or neurological illness.

These conditions may not preclude you from practicing yoga or increasing the difficulty of your routine, but you might need to avoid certain poses or modify others. The Get Active Questionnaire (GAQ), a tool developed by the Canadian Society for Exercise Physiology, can also help you determine whether you should talk to your doctor before embarking on, or ramping up, any fitness or flexibility program. You can find it at www.health.harvard.edu/GAQ.

If you do need to speak to a doctor, show him or her this report—or provide pictures of any other poses that you're thinking of trying. He or she may be able to say whether specific poses would be either beneficial or harmful for you, or even recommend an instructor, class, or studio. If you are taking a yoga class, talk to the instructor before class about your limitations.

Advice for people with arthritis

Yoga can help ease arthritis by increasing your range of motion and improving flexibility. The feel-good hormones that yoga promotes can also help alleviate the stress that often increases pain. Still, it's wise to exercise a few basic cautions.

Go easy. You should steer clear of vigorous practices that may aggravate already damaged joints.

Keep moving. A gentle Vinyasa or flow class may be preferable to a class where postures are held for longer periods of time. Holding static postures may be painful for some people with arthritis. If this is a problem for you, gently move in and out of a posture

▶ Red flags that warrant a call to 911

Yoga is unlikely to trigger serious problems like a stroke or heart attack. But if you experience any of the following symptoms during or after yoga, call 911:

- piercing pain in the back of the neck
- partial facial paralysis
- chest pain, pressure, heaviness, or tightness
- faintness or loss of consciousness
- significant or persistent shortness of breath or dizziness.

Ask your doctor whether any other warning signs specific to your health history warrant a call. You should also call your doctor if a routine you've been doing for a while without discomfort starts to cause you pain.

even if the rest of the class is holding it. For example, instead of holding still in warrior II pose (see page 22), gently bend and straighten your front knee. It's best to let the instructor know ahead of time that you have arthritis and might need to do this.

Delay your practice until later in the day. With some types of arthritis (such as rheumatoid arthritis), joints tend to be stiffer in the morning. Waiting until later in the day allows your muscles and joints to loosen up. Only you can tell when yoga will feel the best for you. Pay attention to your body, and practice yoga at the time of day that feels most appropriate.

Check with your doctor about flare-ups. When your joints are hurting, you may still be able to do yoga, but for a shorter length of time or at a lower intensity than usual. This can help keep your joints mobile. Talk to your doctor about what's right for you. And remember, you could always do some breathing exercises and meditations instead of postures.

Advice for people with high blood pressure

Research suggests that regular practice of yoga can help to lower high blood pressure. But when you do any type of exercise, including yoga, your blood pressure tends to rise in the short term. Here's how to keep it under control when you're on the mat.

Choose middle ground. Vigorous practices, as well as more static ones in which you are holding poses for longer periods of time, can raise blood pressure. To minimize any spikes, move gently from one pose to the next, and move within a pose if it is being held for more than 10 seconds. (See "Keep moving," page 13, for an example.)

Rest more. Just because the class is still holding downward-facing dog doesn't mean you have to. Simply bring your knees down to the mat and rest in child's pose. Taking rest breaks between moves will help to keep your blood pressure lower.

Don't hold your breath. Holding your breath can cause your blood pressure to spike. Instead, remind yourself to keep breathing. Also, don't strain to lengthen your inhalations and exhalations or force your chest or abdomen to expand as you inhale.

Keep your head up. Inverted postures, like head or shoulder stands, are risky moves for many. They also cause significant rises in blood pressure.

Make meditation mandatory. This is done at the end of class, sometimes while lying in corpse pose (*savasana*). If your blood pressure has gone up during your practice, relaxing at the end slows your body down and lowers blood pressure and breathing rate.

Advice for people with osteoporosis

There is emerging evidence that yoga postures may help keep bones strong. For one study, 30 postmenopausal women with osteoporosis took classes four days a week for six months. At the end, their bone density had increased somewhat. However, certain yoga moves may be risky if you have a severe case.

Flex forward with caution. When you do standing or seated forward bends, knees-to-chest, or cat-cow, you are performing forward spinal flexion. The front part of the spine is compressed during this type of movement, which may increase risk of fractures if you have severe osteoporosis. If you already have a compression fracture, you should avoid forward bends completely.

Check with your doctor before doing side bends and twists. These actions compress the spine and may increase the risk of a spinal fracture, too.

Advice for people with glaucoma

This eye condition results in damage to the optic nerve because of elevated pressure in the eye, so the last thing you want to do is increase pressure in your eyes, as certain yoga postures can do.

Keep your head up. Postures in which your head is down—such as head and shoulder stands, downward-facing dog, and forward bends—increase pressure inside the eye, which may raise the risk of glaucoma progression. In one study, even the legs-up-the-wall pose increased pressure inside the eye.

Don't hold your breath. Just as it increases blood pressure, it may raise pressure inside your eyes.

Stop a pose immediately if you experience sudden eye pain, or if you develop a headache, blurred vision, or the appearance of halos around lights. ♥

How to use the yoga practices in this report

In this report, you will find six routines. The Basic Practice is the foundation of the program. In addition, there are five add-on routines—the Flexibility Practice, Balance Practice, Strengthening Practice, Energizing Practice, and Calming Practice—that you can use in conjunction with the Basic Practice to further specific goals.

To start with, concentrate on the Basic Practice, as everything else that follows builds on that routine. After a week or two, once you know the poses and flows in that routine well enough to do them without having to read the descriptions any more, choose a goal that you want to work on and try the corresponding practice. If you are feeling stressed, you might want to try the Calming Practice. If you're feeling sluggish after sitting all day at work, the Energizing Practice might be just what you need. You can stick with one routine for a few weeks, or change it up based on how you're feeling or what you need that day.

As you will see, the Basic Practice begins with a sequence called the ten churnings (page 18), which limbers up all of the major joints. If you don't have time for a full routine, you can use the ten churnings as a mini routine at any point throughout the day.

Whatever mix you choose, aim to do some yoga every day.

Equipment

One of the beauties of yoga is that you don't need a lot of expensive equipment or clothing. The following basics are considered standard and are helpful for these routines:

- A flat space. That means a space that's large enough for you to stretch out on the floor and high enough for you to reach your arms over your head.
- A comfortable, nonskid surface. A yoga mat can help prevent you from slipping as you hold postures. However, if you're practicing on a carpet at home, the carpet may do the trick—and provide cushioning as well—so you can skip the mat. If you need more cushioning, another option is to substitute a traditional gym mat for a yoga mat.
- Loose, comfortable clothes. That means loose or stretchy pants and a top that allows freedom of movement. You don't want anything restrictive.

The following optional pieces will help you modify moves to meet your personal needs:

- Strap. The strap gives your arms a bit more reach in certain poses or stretches. You can buy a cotton yoga strap online, but a belt or the tie from your bathrobe will work, too.
- Pillows, blankets, bolster, blocks, or towels. These

How does yoga fit in to your exercise regimen?

The Physical Activity Guidelines for Americans recommend at least 150 minutes of moderate-intensity aerobic physical activity (the kind that gets your heart rate up) in addition to twice-weekly strength-training sessions, plus balance exercises for those who need them. So where does yoga fit in?

While the guidelines and the American Heart Association say that some forms of yoga can be vigorous enough to get your heart rate up, the routines in this report are unlikely to elicit such a change. So along with your yoga practice, be sure to get some cardio exercise, such as walking, biking, or playing tennis.

As for muscle strengthening, a number of the postures in the routines—such as downward-facing dog (page 21), chair pose (page 38), and half boat pose (page 40)—may help to make your muscles stronger, especially when you first begin. It would be reasonable to count any of the routines here toward the muscle-strengthening recommendations in the guidelines. However, you may want to supplement with activities like lifting weights, especially as the yoga moves become easier. You need to keep challenging your muscles.

Yoga can also help with balance and avoiding falls. The Balance Practice is the best for helping to improve your stability.

can provide support when you are holding certain positions such as a bridge or child's pose.

Terminology used in the routines

As you'll see, our instructions include some specific terminology, as follows:

Repetitions (reps). Each rep is a single, complete performance of a movement or posture.

Hold. This tells you the number of breaths to take while maintaining a posture. Start with a comfortable number of breaths, then work up.

Starting position. This describes how to position your body before starting the movement.

Movement. This explains how to assume a pose or perform one complete rep of a flow.

Tips and techniques. We offer a few pointers to help you maintain good form and avoid injury.

Make it easier. If you have trouble performing an exercise, this option makes it less difficult.

Tips for a better, safer practice

To reap the most benefit from the routines in this report and avoid injuries, here are a few points to keep in mind as you go through the poses. (Also see "Avoiding injuries in class," page 52, if you move on to organized classes or follow programs online.)

Maintain proper form and alignment. Good posture and alignment count for a lot when you're doing yoga and can help you avoid injuries. Good alignment generally means keeping your body in a straight line from head to toe except for the slight natural curves of the spine. However, proper alignment varies by pose. Try to maintain the same form as pictured for each of the poses, and carefully follow the instructions, especially the tips and techniques. If you are unable to execute a posture with good form, don't go as deep into it. For example, place your hands on a chair or your leg instead of the floor, or don't bend your knees as much.

When instructions in our routines ask you to stand or sit up straight, that means
- chin parallel to the floor
- arms at your sides, elbows relaxed and even
- shoulders even (roll them up, back, and down to help achieve this)
- abdominal muscles pulled in
- hips even
- knees even and pointing straight ahead
- feet pointing straight ahead
- body weight evenly distributed on both feet when standing.

Don't slouch. If you can't sit erect on the floor, sit on the edge of a folded-up blanket or in a chair. Slouching puts more load on your spine, which may aggravate osteoporosis or other problems in the back.

Pay attention to your breathing. In addition to the separate breathing techniques for each practice, try to coordinate your breath with the movements, as you move into and out of yoga postures or through a series of postures. This coordination establishes a deeper, more regular breathing pattern that enhances relaxation. You will find specific directions in the instructions for each routine.

Go for "aahh," not "ouch." Yoga should never hurt. You should move into a posture to the point where it feels like a pleasant stretch. Challenge yourself, but avoid strain. If a posture hurts, stop immediately. Reset your positioning and try again. If it still hurts, modify the move so it is comfortable for you.

Keep the movements slow and controlled. Move in and out of poses slowly and as smoothly as possible for a more meditative practice and to avoid injury. Avoid thrusting or jerking movements.

Get up slowly. Moving from lying down to sitting or from sitting to standing can cause blood pressure to drop, resulting in dizziness. The cause is a temporary reduction in blood flow inside the skull and thus a temporary shortage of oxygen to the brain. This problem becomes more common as you age. To prevent it, take extra time to get up. If you are lying on the floor, roll onto your side and slowly sit up. From that seated position, get on your feet and slowly rise, rolling up one vertebra at a time with your head coming up last.

Keep it complementary. Do not use yoga to replace conventional medical care or to postpone seeing a health care provider about pain or any other medical condition.

Basic Practice

The Basic Practice is an intermediate-level routine that forms the foundation of this program. You should aim to do the practice three times a week for full benefits; however, you can also do it daily if you like.

Once you're comfortable with this routine—usually after about two weeks of consistent practice—you can tailor your practice by choosing one of the specialized routines that follow. Each one integrates new postures into the Basic Practice in order to achieve a certain goal: increasing flexibility, improving balance, building strength, boosting your energy, or restoring calm. You can focus on one specialized routine for as many weeks as you want, or switch from one to the next depending on how you are feeling on a given day. But it helps to be very familiar with the Basic Practice before moving to the specialized ones, because we do not repeat the instructions for each pose later on; we give only the name of each pose and sometimes a thumbnail photo as a quick reminder. You can also do the Basic Practice by itself at any time.

The Basic Practice begins with a deep breathing exercise, followed by the ten churnings and then a series of postures. You'll end with some relaxation and meditation. The routine will take about 30 to 45 minutes to complete.

➤ Three-part breath

Sit comfortably with your spine elongated. Place your right palm on or just above your navel. As you inhale through your nose, notice your belly pressing against your palm. As you exhale, notice your belly easing away from your palm. Repeat 3 times.

Keeping your right palm on your belly, place your left palm on the left side of your rib cage. As you inhale through your nose, notice your rib cage pressing against your palm. As you exhale, feel your ribcage easing away from your palm. Repeat 3 times.

Keeping your left palm on your ribcage, place your right palm on your upper chest. As you inhale through your nose, notice your chest rising against your palm. As you exhale, feel your chest easing away from your palm. Repeat 3 times.

Release your hands down and see if you can feel your belly, ribcage, and chest rise as you inhale and lower as you exhale. Close your eyes if you like. Breathe slowly. Repeat 3 to 6 times. (For a video demonstration, go to www.health.harvard.edu/three-part-breath.)

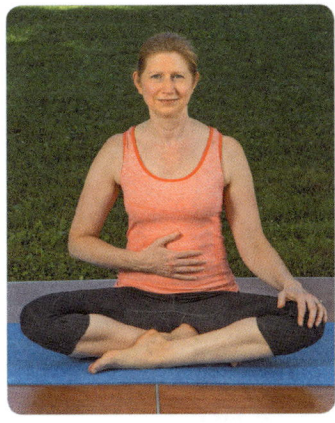 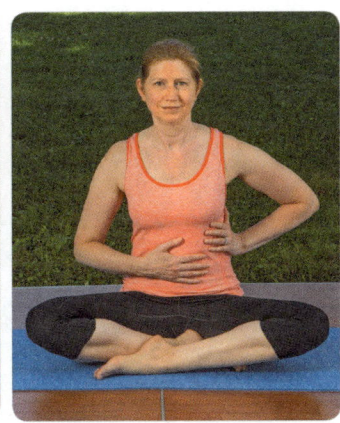 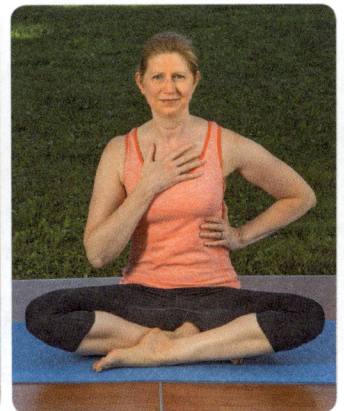 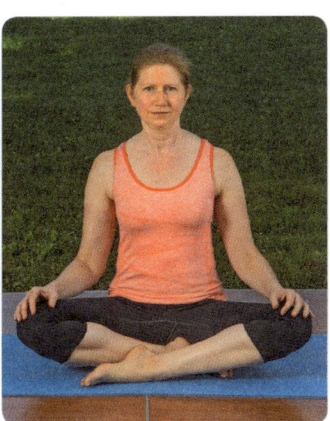

Special thanks to **Laura Malloy**, a certified yoga teacher, yoga therapist and one of the editors of this report, for demonstrating the exercises and stretches illustrated here.

Basic Practice

➤ Ten churnings

The churnings loosen up your joints and serve as a warm-up. Do each one 10 times in both directions and then repeat on the opposite side when applicable. This routine can be done on its own to help you get moving in the morning or to counteract stiffness after sitting for too long. (For a video demonstration, go to www.health.harvard.edu/ten-churnings.)

1. Right ankle circles

Stand with your right foot behind you with just your toes on the floor, arms relaxed at your sides. Rotate your ankle clockwise 10 times, then repeat in the opposite direction, circling your ankle counterclockwise.

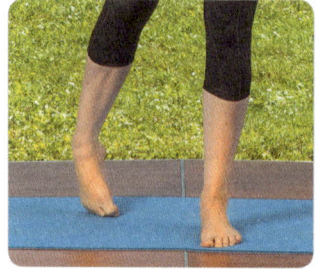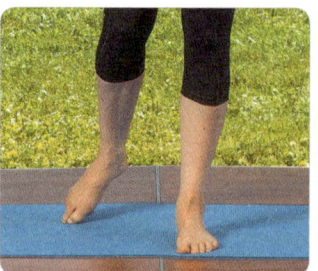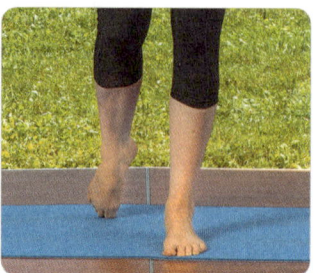

2. Left ankle circles

Switch feet and repeat the ankle circles, with your left foot back.

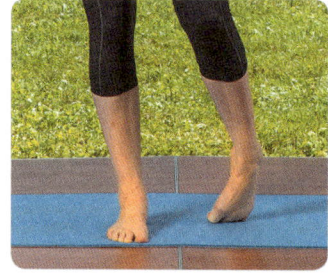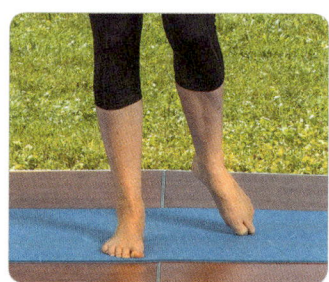

3. Head circles

Stand with your feet hip-width apart, arms relaxed at your sides. Rotate your head 10 times clockwise as if you're drawing a circle with your nose in front of you. Repeat counterclockwise.

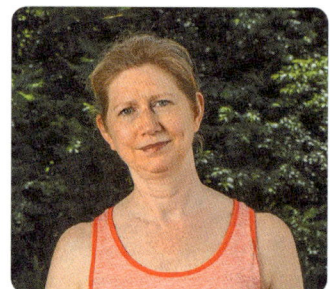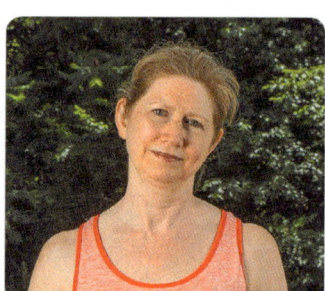

4. Shoulder circles

Stand with your feet hip-width apart, arms relaxed at your sides. Roll your shoulders up, back, and then down 10 times. Let your arms follow, keeping them relaxed and elbows slightly bent. Repeat in the opposite direction.

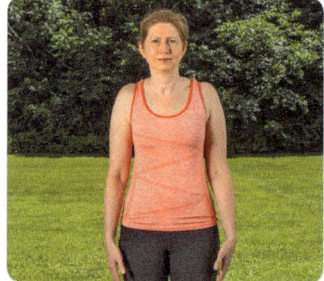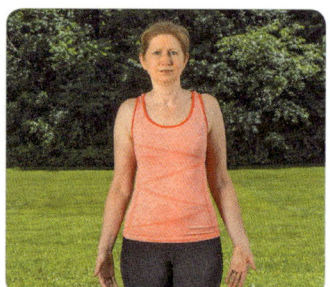

5. Wrist circles

Stand with your arms in front of you with your fingers interlaced and your forearms together. Rotate your hands and wrists 10 times clockwise, keeping your elbows and upper arms stationary. Repeat counterclockwise.

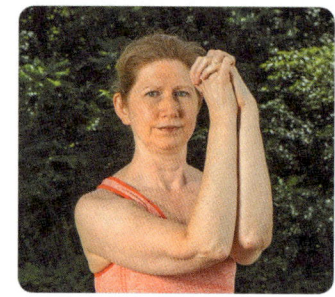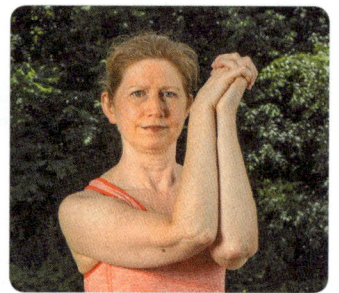

6. Side stretches

Stand with your feet hip-width apart, arms at your sides with your hands in loose fists. Bend at your waist to your right, raising your left arm up toward your left armpit while your right arm slides down your leg. Repeat to the opposite side. Do 10 to each side.

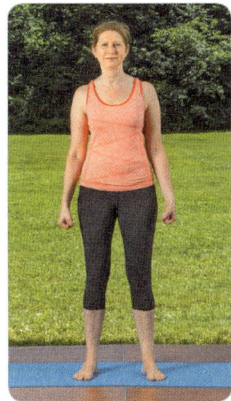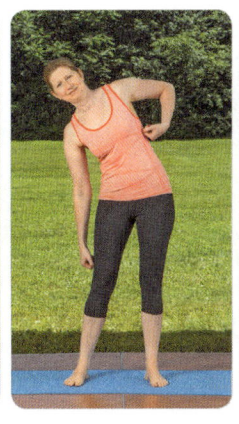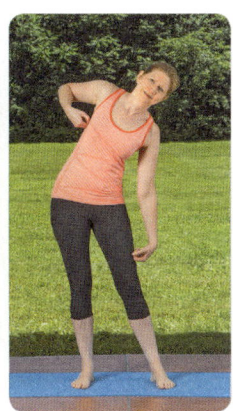

7. Twists

Stand with your feet a little wider than hip-width apart, arms relaxed at your sides. Turn your upper body to the right and look over your right shoulder, as your left hand swings toward your right shoulder and your right arm bends behind you. Repeat turning to the left, and continue alternating sides. Keep your hips and legs facing forward. Do 10 to each side.

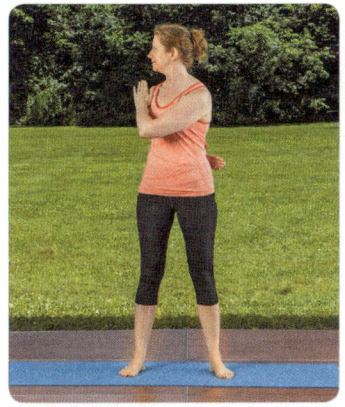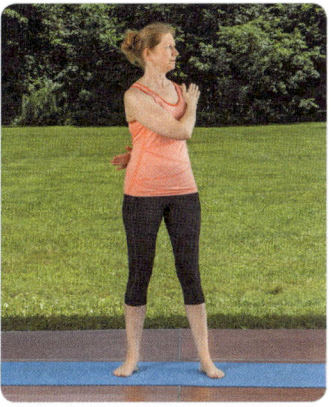

8. Hip circles

Stand with your feet a little wider than hip-width apart, arms relaxed at your sides. Rotate your hips 10 times clockwise, keeping your spine and legs straight. Imagine you're a wooden spoon stirring a pot. You should feel it in the tops of your thighs at your hip sockets. Repeat counterclockwise.

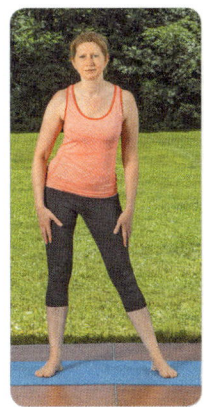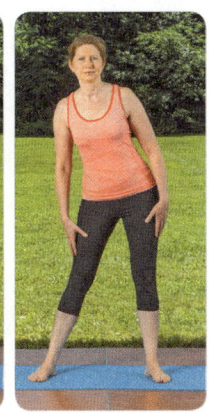

9. Knee circles

Stand with your feet and legs together, bend your knees slightly, and place your hands on your knees or thighs. Circle your knees 10 times clockwise. You'll also get some rotation in your ankles. Repeat counterclockwise.

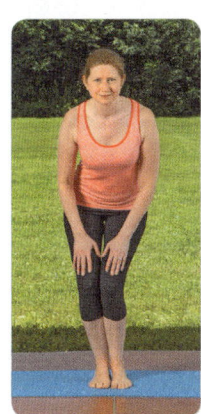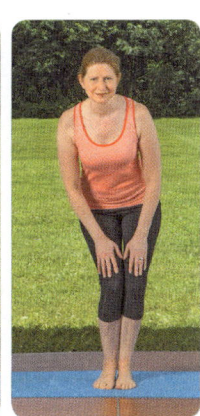

10. Spine ripples

Stand with your feet hip-width apart and bend your knees slightly. Lift your tailbone behind you, and then bring it forward and let the movement flow up your entire spine like a wave. Let your arms swing naturally. Repeat for a total of 10 times.

Tips and techniques for all 10 churnings:
- Keep the movements slow and controlled.
- Let your breath flow slowly and smoothly.

Make it easier: Do fewer reps, make the movements smaller, or do them more slowly.

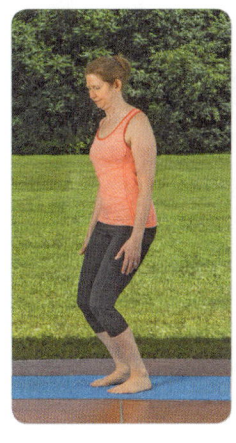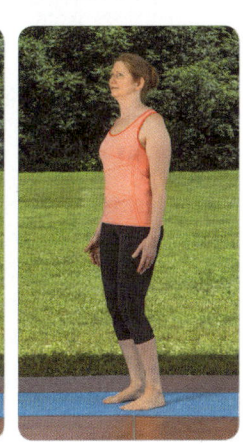

Basic Practice

➤ Mountain pose

Starting position: Stand tall with your feet slightly apart. Relax your arms at your sides with your shoulders back and down.

Movement: There is no actual movement in this pose, but your muscles are actively engaged. Imagine your feet are rooted in the ground, and draw your fingertips down toward the floor. At the same time, draw your head toward the ceiling, elongating your body.

Where you'll feel it: Entire body

Hold: 3 to 6 slow, easy breaths

Reps: 1

Tips and techniques:
- Don't arch or round your back.
- Don't hold your breath.
- Engage your abdominal muscles to support your back.

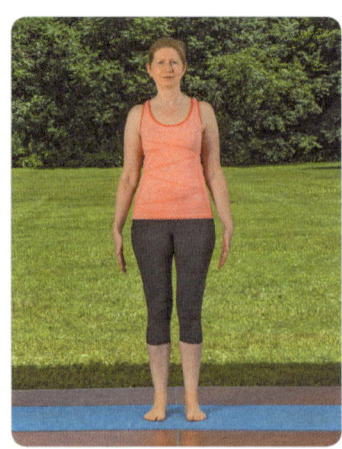

➤ Half sun salutation

Starting position: Mountain pose.

Movement: This exercise is called a flow, because you're moving from one asana to another rather than performing each one as a separate exercise. From mountain pose (**A**), you move as follows (for a video demonstration, go to www.health.harvard.edu/half-sun-salutation):

Upward salute (B): As you inhale, turn your palms away from you and raise your arms out to the sides and then overhead.

Forward fold (C): As you exhale, fold forward from your hips, bringing your arms down out to the side, then down toward the floor.

Half forward fold (D): Inhale and lift your head and chest, flattening your back and letting your hands slide up your shins. (This is also called a half fold.)

Forward fold (E): Exhale and return to the full forward fold.

Upward salute (F): Inhale as you stand back up, bringing your arms out to the sides and then overhead.

Mountain pose (G): Exhale as you lower your arms back to the starting position.

Where you'll feel it: Entire body

Reps: 3

Tips and techniques:
- Keep the movement slow and controlled.
- Keep your shoulders relaxed and down, away from your ears.
- Move within a comfortable range of motion. Do not strain or force any position.
- Engage your abdominal muscles to support your back.

Make it easier: Place your hands on your thighs or a chair for the forward fold.

If you have back problems or osteoporosis, check with your doctor before doing this flow.

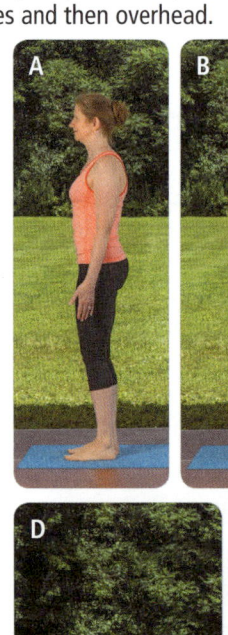
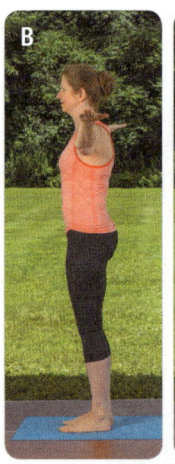
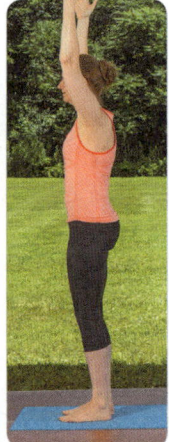
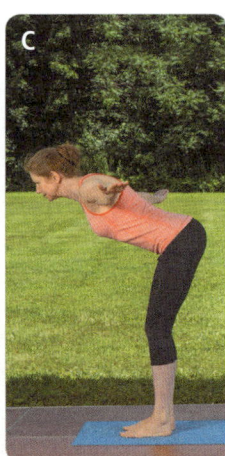
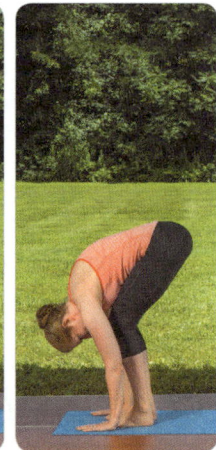
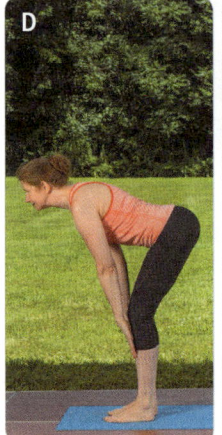
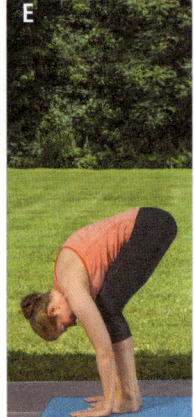
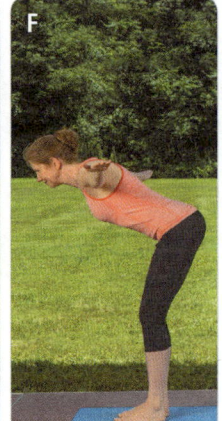
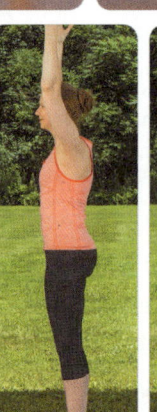
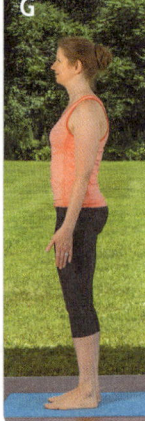

➤ Sun salutation

Starting position: Mountain pose (**A**).

Movement: Start with a half sun salutation—upward salute (**B**), forward fold (**C**), half forward fold (**D**), forward fold (**E**)—but do not return to standing. Instead, continue the flow as follows (for a video, go to www.health.harvard.edu/full-sun-salutation):

Lunge (F): Place your hands flat on the floor. Inhale as you step your right foot back into a deep lunge.

Plank (G): Exhale as you step your left foot back to meet your right foot. Your shoulders should be directly over your hands, and your body should be in a straight line from head to heels. Hold.

Child's pose (H): Inhale and lower knees to the floor. As you exhale, sit back onto your heels, lower your forehead to the floor, and extend your arms in front of you. Hold for 3 breaths.

Upward-facing dog (I): From child's pose, shift your weight forward onto your hands and lie facedown with your legs extended behind you and toes pointed. Place your hands, palms down, on the floor by your chest with your elbows pointing behind you. Pressing into your hands and the tops of your feet, inhale and lengthen your spine toward the ceiling, lifting your torso and thighs off the floor. Balance on your palms and tops of your feet.

Downward-facing dog (J): Exhale and tuck your toes, shifting your weight to the balls of your feet; then press into your hands and the balls of the feet, as you lift your hips toward the ceiling, forming an inverted V. Hold 3 to 6 breaths.

Lunge (K): Inhale as you step your right foot forward in between your hands.

Forward fold (L): On an exhale, bring your left foot alongside your right foot and bend forward from the hips.

End with the rest of a half sun salutation—half forward fold (**M**), forward fold (**N**), upward salute (**O**), and mountain pose (**P**).

Repeat the entire sequence on the other side, stepping back into the lunge with your left foot. This completes one rep.

Continued on page 22

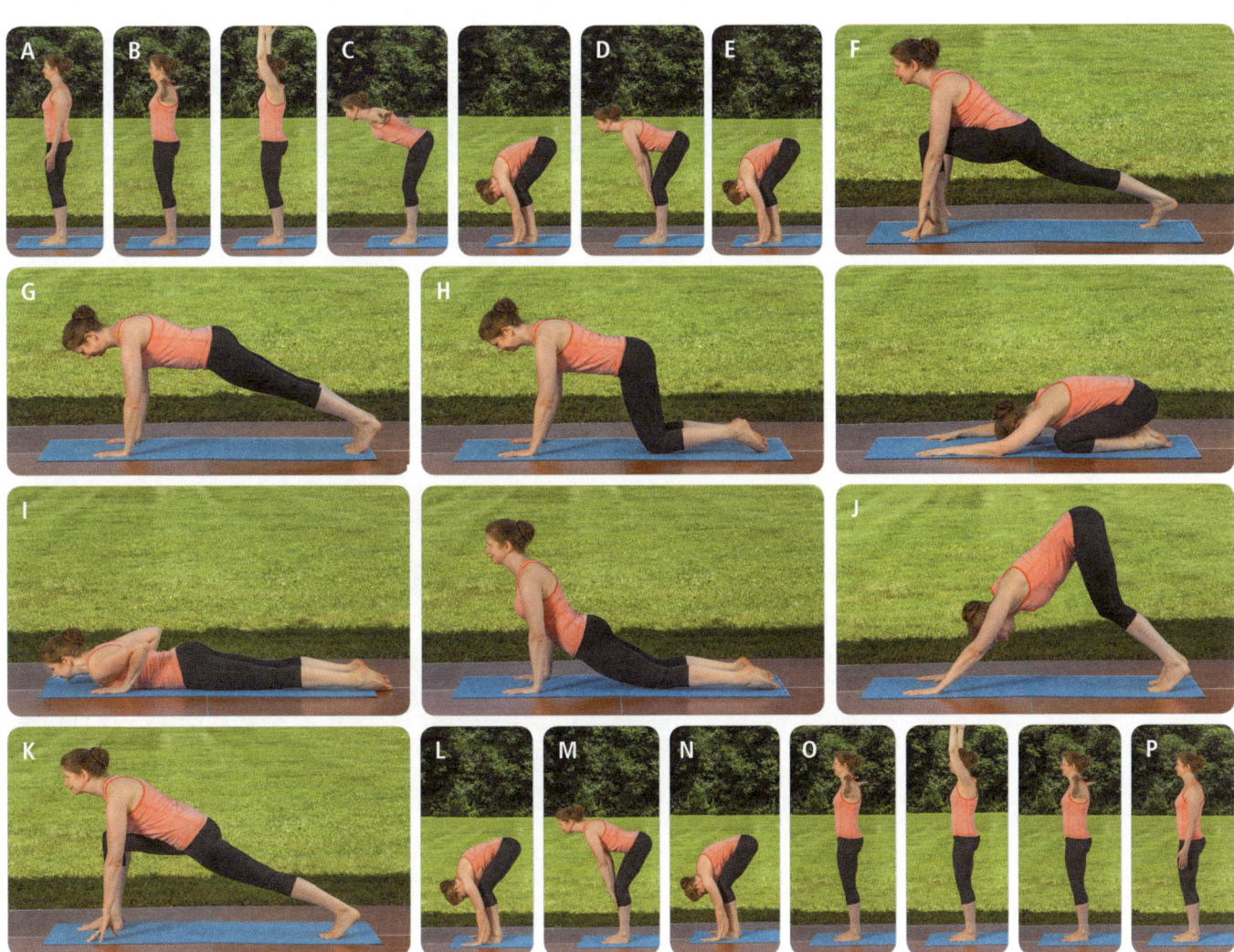

Basic Practice

Continued from page 21

Where you'll feel it: Entire body

Reps: 1

Tips and techniques:
- Keep the movement slow and controlled.
- Keep your shoulders relaxed and down, away from your ears.
- Move within a comfortable range of motion. Do not strain or force any position.

- Engage your core muscles to support your back.

Make it easier: Place your knee(s) on the floor for the lunge, plank, or downward-facing dog. Place your hands on your thighs or a chair for the forward fold. Don't lift as high for upward-facing dog.

If you have back problems or osteoporosis, check with your doctor before doing this flow.

➤ Tree pose

Note: This pose and the next four poses—warrior II, reverse warrior, side angle, and triangle pose—form a sequence. Do this sequence starting with the right foot. Later you will repeat the sequence starting with the left foot.

Starting position: Mountain pose.

Movement: As you inhale, raise your right foot off the floor and place it on the inside of your left thigh, with your right leg turned outward and your right knee pointing toward the side. Raise your arms into prayer pose in front of your body. When you are sure of your balance, raise your arms overhead. Hold. Return to mountain pose on an exhale.

Where you'll feel it: Entire body

Hold: 3 to 6 slow, easy breaths

Reps: 1

Tips and techniques:
- Look at a stationary spot at eye level to help you balance.

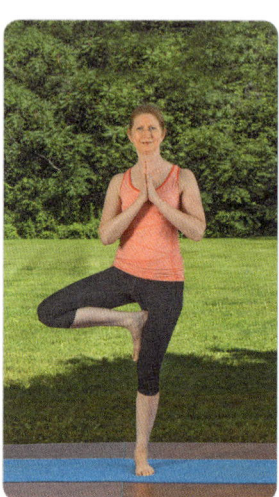 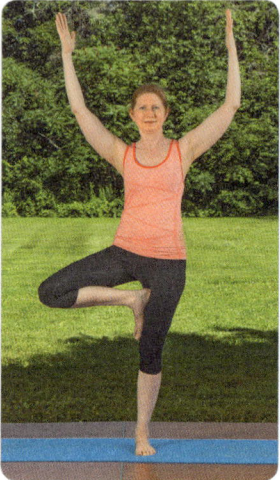 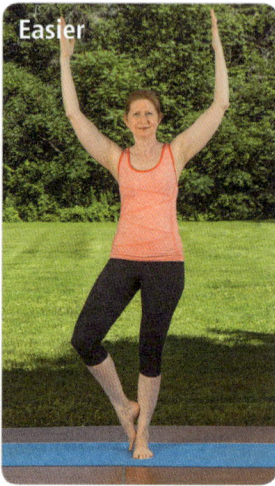

- Don't arch or round your back.
- Don't place your foot on the opposite knee.
- Keep your shoulders relaxed and down, away from your ears.
- Engage your abdominal muscles to stand tall and support your back.

Make it easier: Place your right foot by your left ankle, keeping your toes on the floor.

➤ Warrior II

Starting position: Move to the top (short side) of the mat and stand in mountain pose, facing the end of the mat.

Movement: On an exhale, step your right foot back, keeping your left foot facing forward. As you inhale, raise your arms to shoulder height, palms down. As you exhale, bend your left knee to align it over your left ankle. Look over the fingers of your left hand. Hold.

Where you'll feel it: Legs, buttocks, back, shoulders, arms

Hold: 3 to 6 slow, easy breaths

Reps: 1

Tips and techniques:
- Imagine that your fingertips are reaching to opposite walls.

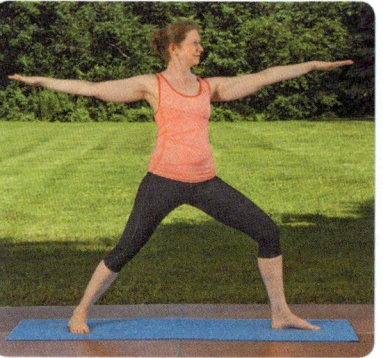 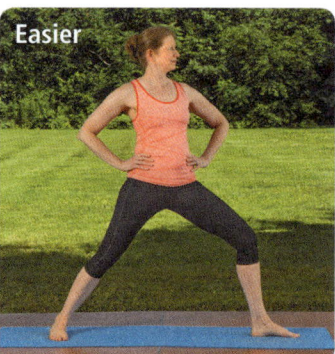

- Keep your hips and shoulders aligned and facing to the right (the long side of your mat).

Make it easier: Place your hands on your hips. Don't lower as far down.

Basic Practice

➤ Reverse warrior

Starting position: Warrior II.

Movement: On an inhale, rotate your left arm so your palm is up and raise your left arm overhead, reaching toward the ceiling and curving it back slightly. At the same time, lower your right arm to your right leg and gaze down toward your right foot. Hold.

Where you'll feel it: Legs, buttocks, back, side of torso, shoulders, arms

Hold: 3 to 6 slow, easy breaths

Reps: 1

Tips and techniques:
- Keep your front knee over your ankle.
- Imagine that your fingertips are reaching to the ceiling.
- Keep your back leg strong.

Make it easier: Keep your arms down with your hands on your thighs.

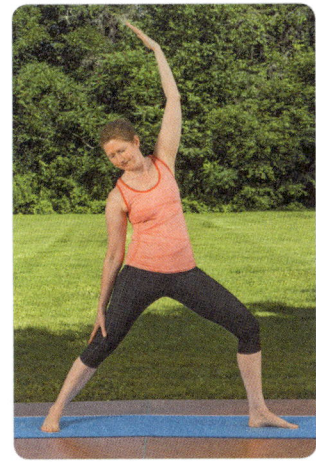
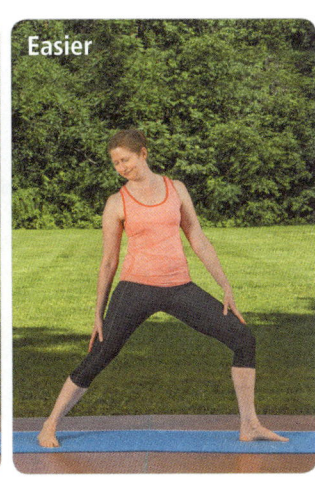

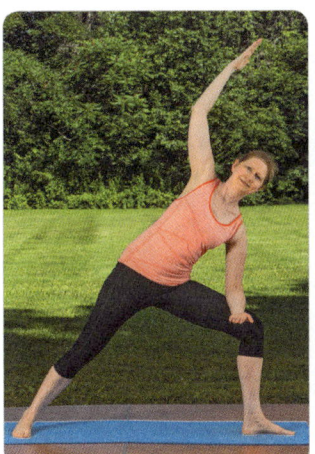
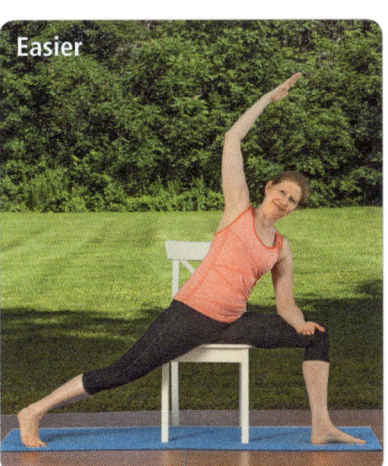

➤ Side angle

Starting position: Reverse warrior.

Movement: Inhale and place your left forearm on your left thigh. Exhale and reach with your right arm overhead toward the left. Hold. Inhale as you return to Warrior II position.

Where you'll feel it: Legs, buttocks, back, side of torso, shoulders, arms

Hold: 3 to 6 slow, easy breaths

Reps: 1

Tips and techniques:
- Keep your front knee over your ankle.
- Don't let your top arm and shoulder roll forward; keep both shoulders facing front.
- Engage your abdominal muscles to support your back.

Make it easier: Sit on the edge of a chair as you hold the pose.

➤ Triangle pose

Starting position: Warrior II.

Movement: As you exhale, straighten your legs. As you inhale, reach your left arm and torso to the left as far as possible, then bend to the left and place your left hand on your left leg wherever comfortable. Raise your right arm toward the ceiling and look up at it. Hold. Imagine that your fingertips are reaching toward the ceiling. Inhale as you come up, and exhale as you lower your arms and bring your feet together, returning to Mountain pose.

Where you'll feel it: Legs, buttocks, back, side of torso, shoulders, arms

Hold: 3 to 6 slow, easy breaths

Reps: 1

Tips and techniques:
- Don't let your top hip or shoulder roll forward.
- Engage your abdominal muscles to support your back.
- Place your hand on your hip if holding your arm up becomes tiring.

Make it easier: Place your hand on the seat of chair.

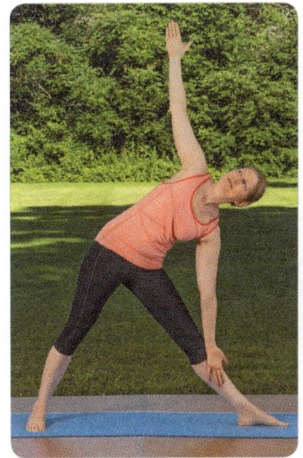
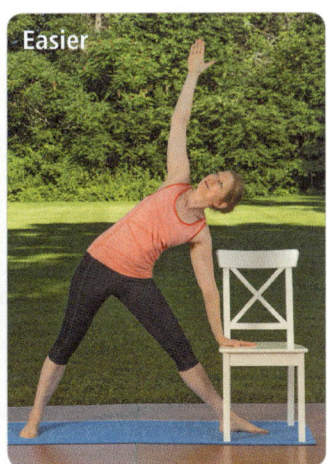

Basic Practice

➤ Repeat the previous sequence on the other side

- Mountain pose
- Tree pose (left foot raised)
- Warrior II (left foot back)
- Reverse warrior (left foot back)
- Side angle (left foot back)
- Triangle pose (left foot back)
- Mountain pose

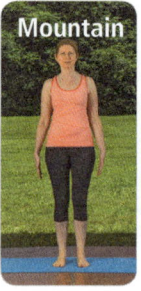
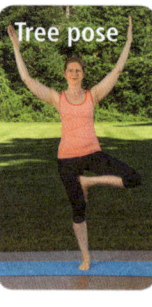
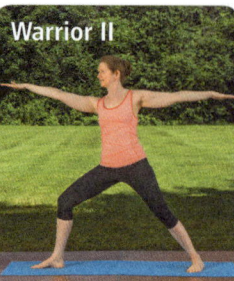
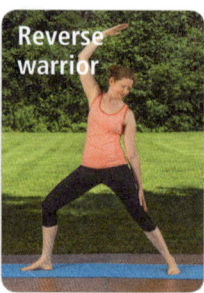
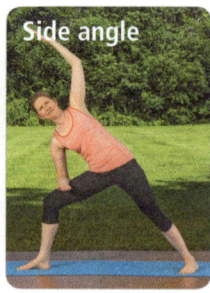
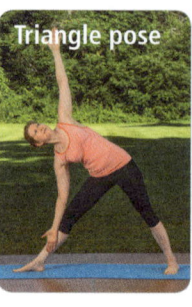
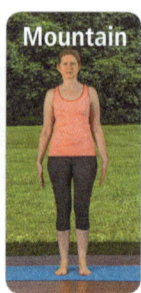

➤ Half sun salutation with downward-facing dog

Starting position: Mountain pose.

Movement: Repeat the half sun salutation sequence—mountain pose (**A**), upward salute (**B**), forward fold (**C**), half forward fold (**D**), forward fold (**E**)—but do not return to standing. Instead, step back into downward-facing dog (**F**). Hold for 3 to 6 breaths. Then lower your knees to the floor (**G**) and sit on the floor (**H**) to prepare for the seated spinal twist (next pose).

Where you'll feel it: Entire body

Reps: 1

Tips and techniques:
- Keep the movement slow and controlled.
- Keep your shoulders relaxed and down, away from your ears.
- Move within a comfortable range of motion. Do not strain or force any position.
- Engage your abdominal muscles to support your back.

Make it easier: Place your hands on your thighs or a chair for the forward fold. For downward-facing dog, keep your knees on the floor or place your hands on a chair.

If you have back problems or osteoporosis, check with your doctor before doing this flow.

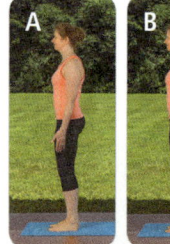
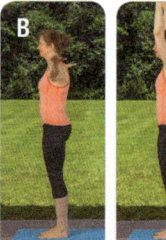
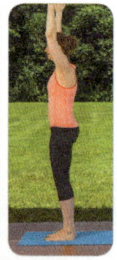
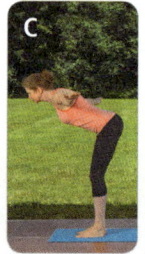
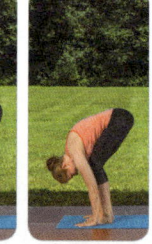
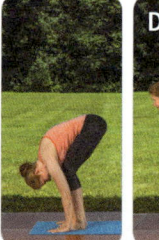
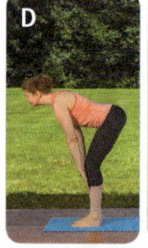
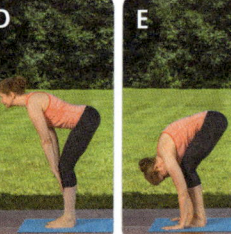
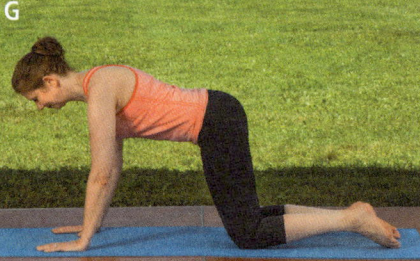
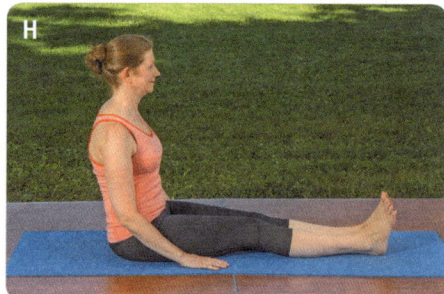

Basic Practice

➤ Seated spinal twist

Starting position: Sit up straight on the floor with your legs together and extended in front of you, feet flexed. Bend your left leg and cross it over your right leg, placing your left foot on the outside of your right thigh. Bend your right (bottom) leg so your right foot is by your left hip. Place your left hand on the floor at your left hip.

Movement: Inhale and sit up tall, extending your spine, and place your right elbow on the outside of your left knee, with your hand pointing upward. Exhale as you rotate your torso toward the left. Hold. Release on an exhale, slowly rotating back to center. Repeat on the opposite side.

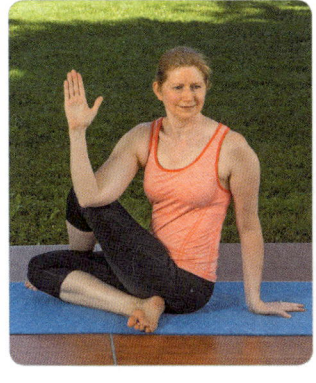

Where you'll feel it: Back, chest, shoulders

Hold: 3 to 6 slow, easy breaths

Reps: 1

Tips and techniques:
- Keep your chest lifted.
- Draw your shoulder blades down your back, away from your ears.

Make it easier: Do a half spinal twist. From the same starting position, twist to the right for a stretch that isn't as deep.

If you have osteoporosis, talk to your doctor before doing this exercise. He or she may recommend a modification or suggest that you avoid it altogether.

➤ Bridge pose

Starting position: Lie faceup with your knees bent and feet flat on the floor. Relax your arms at your sides, palms down.

Movement: As you inhale, lift your buttocks and lower and mid-back off the floor so your knees, hips, and shoulders are in a straight line. Hold. Exhale as you slowly lower.

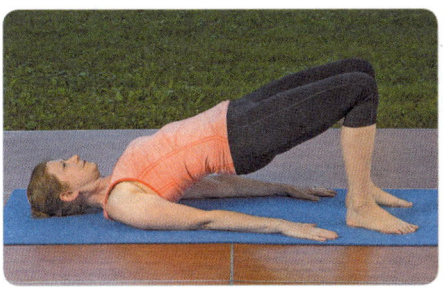
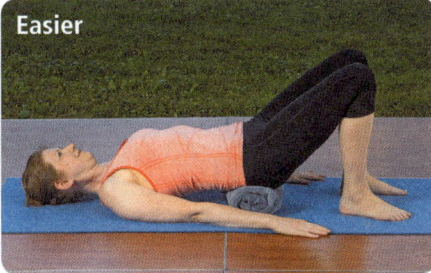

Where you'll feel it: Abdomen, back, buttocks, legs

Hold: 3 to 6 slow, easy breaths

Reps: 1

Tips and techniques:
- Keep your knees in line with your hips and feet, not rolling in or out.
- Lift only to the point where your torso is in line with your knees and shoulders.
- Draw your shoulder blades toward each other.
- Don't hold your breath.

Make it easier: Place a pillow or rolled-up towel under your back for support.

➤ Knees-to-chest

Starting position: Lie faceup with your knees bent and feet flat on the floor.

Movement: On an exhale, bring your knees in toward your chest, grasping your shins. Hold.

Where you'll feel it: Back, hips

Hold: 3 to 6 slow, easy breaths

Reps: 1

Tips and techniques:
- Keep your shoulders down, away from your ears.
- Keep your head on the floor.
- Flex your feet.

Make it easier: Don't pull your knees in as far.

If you have back problems or osteoporosis, or have had surgery recently, check with your doctor before doing this move.

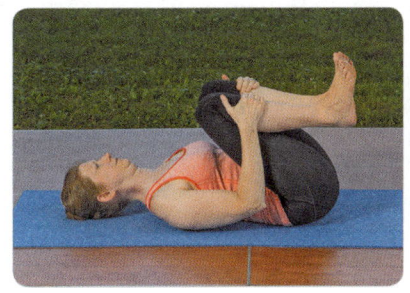
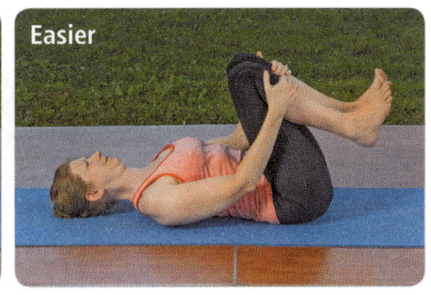

Basic Practice

➤ Wide knee circles

Starting position: Lie on your back, with your knees bent in toward your chest. Spread your knees apart and place a hand on each knee.

Movement: Use your hands to circle your knees away from each other and then toward each other.

Where you'll feel it: Back, hips

Reps: 3 in one direction, then 3 in the other direction

Tips and techniques:
- Keep the movement slow and controlled.
- Don't rock as you circle your knees.
- Keep your shoulders down, away from your ears.
- Keep your head on the floor.

Make it easier: Make smaller circles.

If you have back problems or osteoporosis, or have had surgery recently, check with your doctor before doing this move.

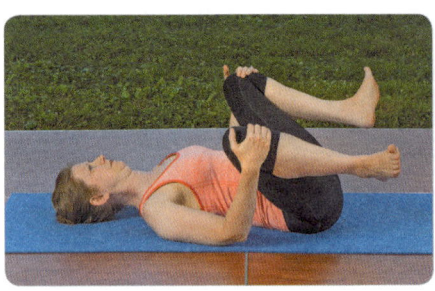
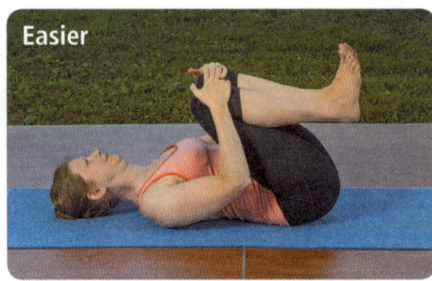

➤ Happy baby pose

Starting position: Lie faceup on the floor with your knees bent.

Movement: Raise the soles of your feet toward the ceiling, keeping your knees bent. With your elbows on the insides of your legs, move your forearms outward over your calves so you can grasp the outer side of each foot. Hold. Release, and lower your feet to the floor.

Where you'll feel it: Back, hips

Hold: 3 to 6 slow, easy breaths

Reps: 1

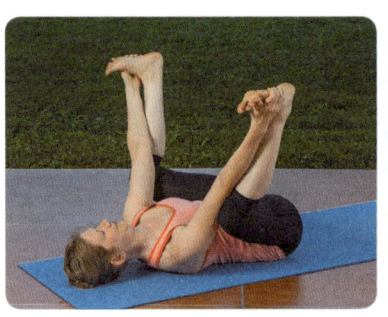
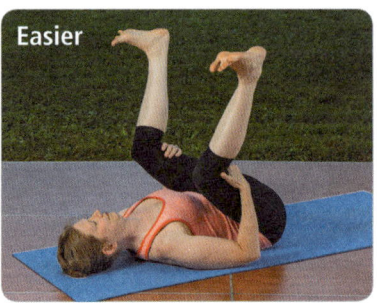

Tips and techniques:
- Keep your shoulders down, away from your ears.
- Keep your head on the floor.

Make it easier: Grasp your calves or thighs.

➤ Lying spinal twist

Starting position: Lie faceup on the floor with your knees bent and feet flat. Extend your arms out to your sides.

Movement: As you exhale, gently lower your knees to the right, keeping both shoulders on the floor. Hold. Return to the center on an inhalation. Repeat on the opposite side.

Where you'll feel it: Back, buttocks, neck

Hold: 3 to 6 slow, easy breaths

Reps: 1

Tips and techniques:
- Keep the movement slow and controlled.
- Move within a comfortable range of motion. Do not strain or force any position.
- Keep your shoulders down, away from your ears.

Make it easier: Extend the lower leg, for greater stability.

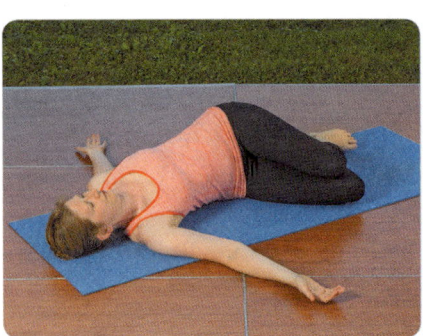
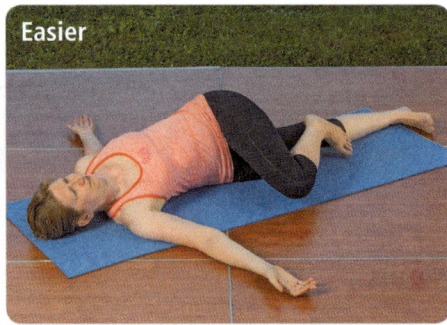

Basic Practice

▸ Corpse pose

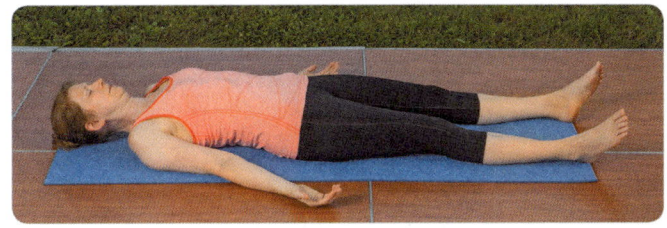

Starting position: Lie on your back with your arms and legs comfortably apart. Palms should be facing up, and your eyes closed. For comfort, you may want to cover yourself with a light blanket. You may also want to cover your eyes with an eye pillow, mask, or towel.

Movement: As you lie on the mat, with your eyes closed, relax each muscle group in turn, starting with your toes and working your way up through your lower and upper legs, buttocks, back, hands, and arms to the top of your head. Take slow, deep breaths, allowing your stomach to rise and fall as you inhale and exhale.

Concentrate on your right big toe and imagine the atoms in it; try to picture the space between the atoms. Imagine your toe feeling warm and relaxed. Repeat on the left. Next, shift your focus to the rest of your toes, then the ball of your foot and the arch.

Work your way up your right leg, turning your attention to your ankle, calf, knee, thigh, and hip. Picture each muscle feeling open, warm, and relaxed. Allow your right leg to relax, sinking into the support of the floor. Repeat on the left side.

Then continue working up to your arms. Is your back feeling tight? Pay attention to the muscles around each vertebra.

Think about your neck and jaw. Allow each part of your face to relax. Let your whole body sink into the floor.

When you are finished, start moving your body gradually to "wake it up": wiggle your fingers and toes, rotate your wrists and ankles, stretch your arms up overhead, and drop your knees to each side to twist the spine. Then roll to one side and sit up slowly to avoid a drop in blood pressure.

Where you'll feel it: Entire body

Hold: 5 minutes to as long as you'd like

Reps: 1

Tips and techniques:
- If your back bothers you, place a bolster or rolled-up towel or blanket under your knees.

▸ Basic breathing meditation

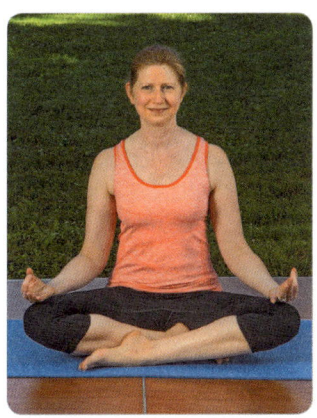

Sit in a comfortable position with an elongated spine, your head erect and your chin slightly tucked in. Position your hands in either wisdom or consciousness mudra (below) and rest them on your thighs. Close your eyes. Begin long, slow deep breathing through your nose. As you inhale, your abdomen should extend as though it is being filled with air. As you continue to inhale, your chest will expand. As you start to exhale, your chest contracts first, followed by your abdomen, which pulls in as though it is being emptied of air. Your breath should be steady and smooth. Focus your attention on the flow of the breath, such as the sound, the temperature of the air in your nostrils, or the movement of your chest and abdomen. Keep your attention on the breath in a relaxed manner. If your attention wanders—which can happen frequently, especially when you're just starting out—patiently and calmly bring your attention back to the breath. Continue for three minutes or longer.

Wisdom and consciousness mudras

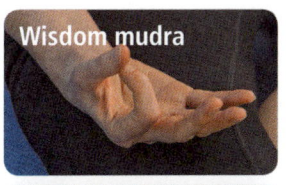

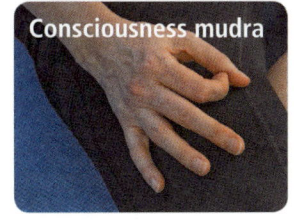

These two mudras use the same finger positions. The difference is whether your palms are facing up or down.

While seated, touch the tip of the index finger to the thumb on each hand. Spread out and extend your other fingers. Rest your hands on your legs. If you are seeking more energy, knowledge, or inspiration from the universe, have your palms facing up toward the sky (wisdom mudra). If you need to calm down or be more grounded, turn your palms to face the earth (consciousness mudra). In both cases, your index finger represents energy from the outside world, while your thumb symbolizes yourself. By forming these two fingers into a circle, you symbolically unite the two.

The wisdom mudra—*gyan mudra* in Sanskrit—is the best known and most widely used hand position among general practitioners of yoga.

Flexibility Practice

Once you've mastered the Basic Practice, you can direct your program by focusing on specific goals. The Flexibility Practice will help you to gain more supple muscles and greater range of motion through various joints. As you advance in your practice, try to think of flexibility in more than just physical terms. While you do this practice, hold the intention in your mind of becoming more adaptable and more accepting of change.

This practice begins with a deep breathing exercise that is unique to this practice. You then perform a number of poses and sequences from the Basic Practice before moving on to some new poses that are specifically aimed at increasing your flexibility. You will continue to alternate various poses from the Basic Practice with new ones from the Flexibility Practice, until you have done all the poses from the Basic Practice, interspersed with new ones. We do not repeat the instructions for each of the exercises from the Basic Practice, so it helps to have learned them first.

You'll finish the routine with some relaxation and meditation. The complete routine will take about 45 to 60 minutes.

➤ Sun breath

Sit comfortably with your spine long. Let your arms rest by your sides. As you inhale through your nose, raise your arms overhead, palms facing each other. As you exhale through your nose, lower your arms back to your sides, palms facing down. Try to coordinate the movement with your breath. Repeat 3 to 6 times. (For a video demonstration, go to www.health.harvard.edu/sun-breath.)

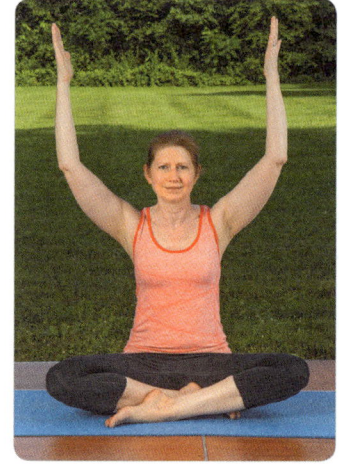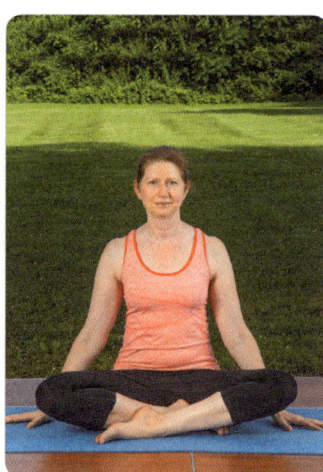

Flexibility Practice

➤ From the Basic Practice

- Ten churnings (right ankle circles, left ankle circles, head circles, shoulder circles, wrist circles, side stretches, twists, hip circles, knee circles, spine ripples)
- Mountain pose
- Half sun salutation (3 times)
- Sun salutation (right foot back; repeat with left foot back; see the photo sequence here if you need a reminder)

Sun salutation

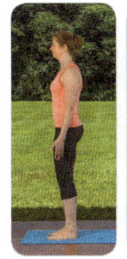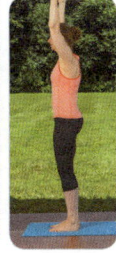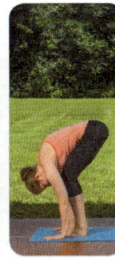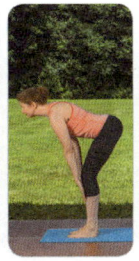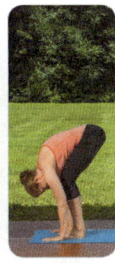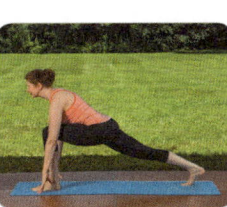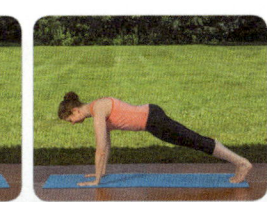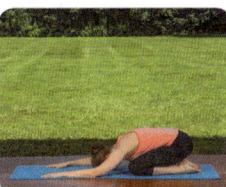

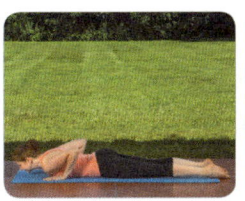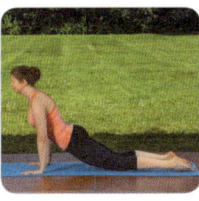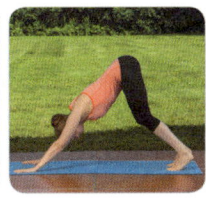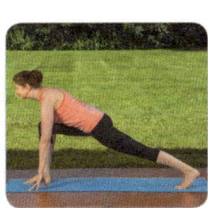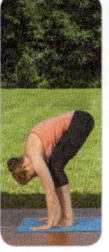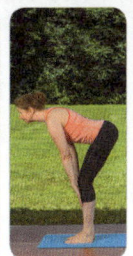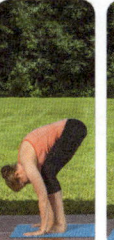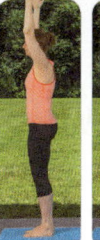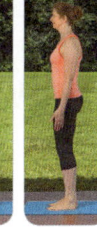

➤ Crescent moon

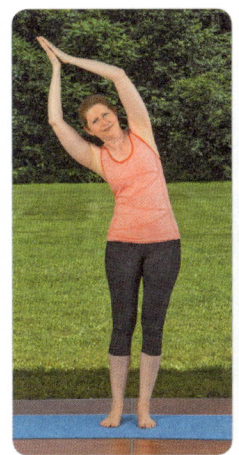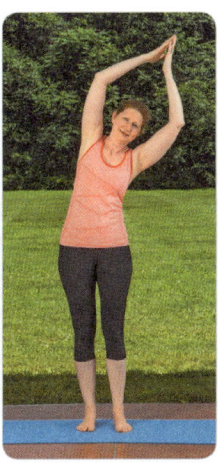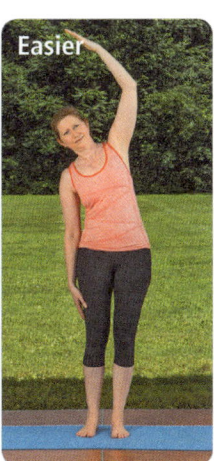

Easier

Starting position: Mountain pose.

Movement: As you inhale, raise your arms out to the sides and overhead, bringing your palms together. Exhale and lean your upper body to the right. Hold. Return to center on an inhale, and then exhale and lean to the left. Hold. Inhale and return to center. Exhale and lower your arms to your sides.

Where you'll feel it: Entire body

Hold: 3 to 6 slow, easy breaths

Reps: 1

Tips and techniques:
- Don't let your top shoulder roll forward; keep your chest open and facing forward.
- Keep your shoulders down and back, away from your ears.
- Engage your abdominal muscles to support your back.

Make it easier: Don't lean as far over. Raise only the arm opposite to the way you are leaning.

Flexibility Practice

➤ From the Basic Practice

- Tree pose (right foot raised)
- Warrior II (right foot back)
- Reverse warrior (right foot back)
- Side angle (right foot back)
- Triangle pose (right foot back)
- Mountain pose

- Tree pose (left foot raised)
- Warrior II (left foot back)
- Reverse warrior (left foot back)
- Side angle (left foot back)
- Triangle pose (left foot back)

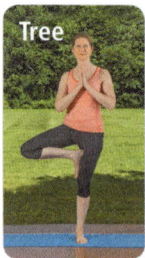
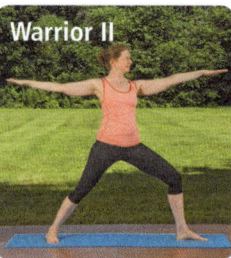
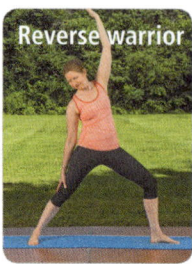
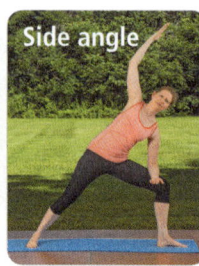
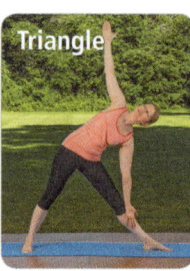
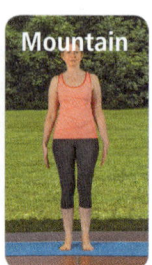

➤ Wide-legged forward fold

Starting position: Stand tall with your feet wider than shoulder-width apart, toes pointing forward. Rest your hands on your hips with your shoulders back and down.

Movement: As you exhale, fold forward from your hips, sliding your hands down the outsides of your legs and then down to the floor. Hold. To flow into the next exercise, do not straighten up again, but bend your knees slightly, bring your feet together, and sit down on the floor.

Where you'll feel it: Back, backs of thighs

Hold: 3 to 6 slow, easy breaths

Reps: 1

Tips and techniques:
- Don't look up; keep your eyes on the floor.
- Keep your shoulders relaxed and down, away from your ears.
- Engage your abdominal muscles to support your back.

Make it easier: Place your hands on your thighs or a chair.

If you have back problems or osteoporosis, check with your doctor before doing this move.

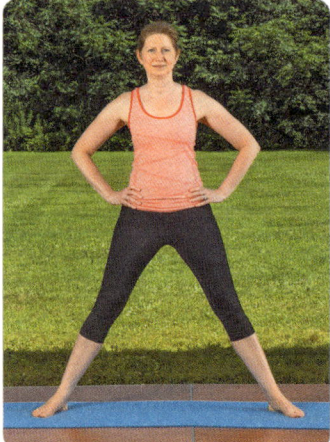
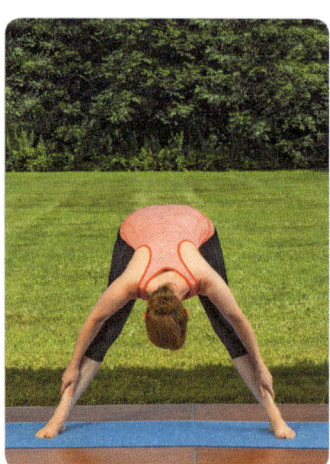
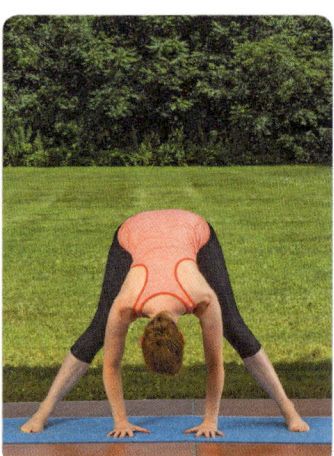

Flexibility Practice

➤ Seated forward fold

Starting position: Sit up straight on the floor with your legs together and extended in front of you, feet flexed. Relax your arms at your sides, hands on the floor.

Movement: Inhale and raise your arms out to the sides and up overhead. As you exhale, lean forward from your hips, reaching your hands toward your feet. Keep your chest lifted and your back neutral. Grasp your feet or your shins, wherever is most comfortable. Hold. On an inhale, release.

Where you'll feel it: Back, backs of thighs

Hold: 3 to 6 slow, easy breaths

Reps: 1

Tips and techniques:
- Don't round your back. If you can't sit up straight, sit on the edge of a rolled-up towel or pillow.
- Draw your shoulder blades down your back, away from your ears.
- Don't let your chin jut forward; keep it slightly tucked.
- Keep your chest lifted.

Make it easier: Loop a strap around your feet and hold on to each end as you lean forward.

If you have back problems or osteoporosis, check with your doctor before doing this move.

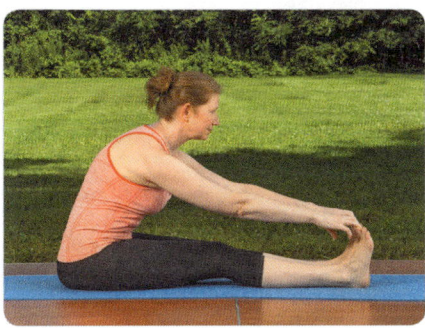
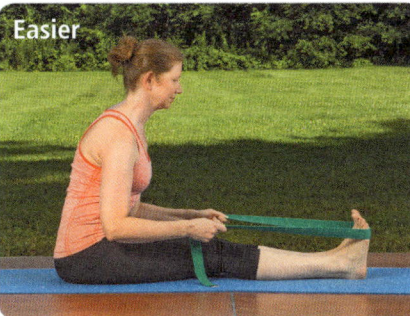

➤ From the Basic Practice

- Seated spinal twist (both sides)

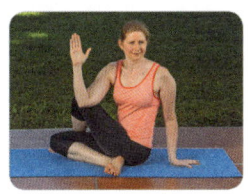

➤ Lying leg stretch

Starting position: Lie on your back on the floor with your knees bent and your feet flat on the floor.

Movement: Grasp the back of your right thigh and straighten your leg so your foot is flexed and your heel is toward the ceiling. Extend your left leg on the floor. Gently pull your right leg toward your chest as far as is comfortable. Hold. Slowly return to the starting position. Repeat on the other side. This is one rep.

Where you'll feel it: Back of thigh

Hold: 3 to 6 slow, easy breaths

Reps: 1

Tips and techniques:
- Keep your leg straight, but don't lock your knee.
- Don't lift your hips off the floor.
- You can bend the leg that you're not stretching and place the foot flat on the floor if that's more comfortable.

Make it easier: Loop a strap around the foot of the leg that you are raising and grasp each end.

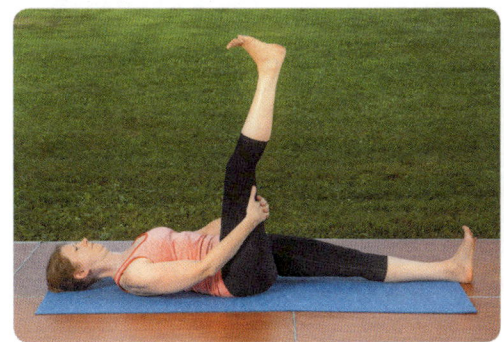
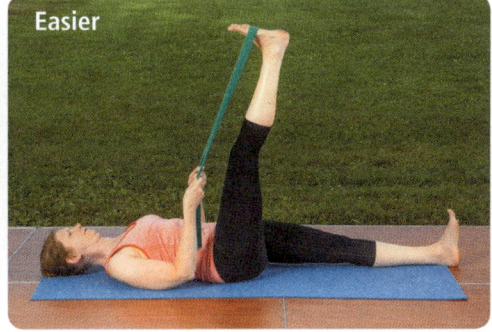

Flexibility Practice

➤ Reclined pigeon

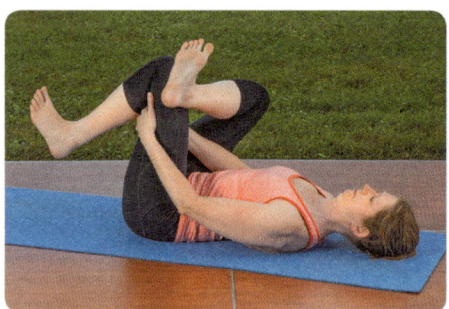 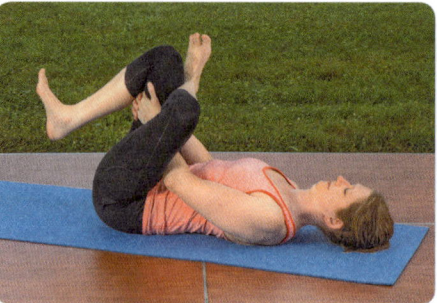 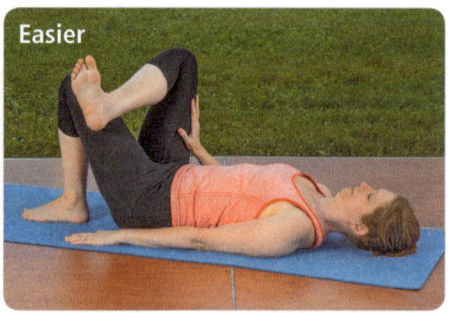

Starting position: Lie on your back with your feet flat on the floor. Cross your right ankle over your left thigh so your right knee is pointing to the right side.

Movement: Grasp the back of your left thigh with both hands and lift your left foot off the floor until you feel a stretch in your right outer hip and buttock. Flex both feet. Hold. Return to the starting position. Repeat on the other side. This is one rep.

Where you'll feel it: Outside of hip and buttocks

Hold: 3 to 6 slow, easy breaths

Reps: 1

Tips and techniques:
- Keep your shoulders back and down, away from your ears.
- Keep your head on the floor.
- Don't roll to the side as you hold this pose.

Make it easier: Keep the left foot on the floor and gently ease the right leg away from you until you feel a stretch.

➤ From the Basic Practice

- Bridge pose
- Knees-to-chest
- Wide knee circles (both directions)
- Happy baby pose
- Lying spinal twist (both sides)
- Corpse pose

Finish with the basic breathing meditation (page 27), using the lotus mudra (below).

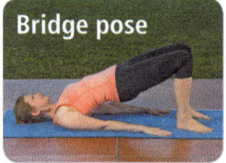 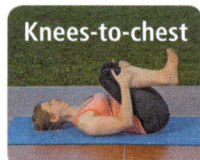 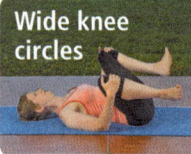 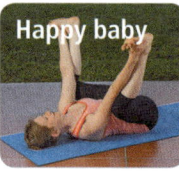 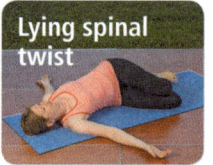 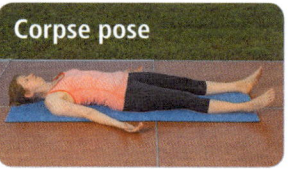

Lotus mudra

Bring the base of your palms together. Press the tips of your thumbs together and do the same with the tips of your pinky fingers. Spread your remaining fingers apart as much as possible. Hold your hands in front of your chest.

This mudra resembles the lotus blossom and symbolizes openness and compassion. Imagine the base of your hands as the plant's strong, sturdy roots and your fingers as the blossom's petals. You can also use this mudra when doing the loving-kindness meditation (see page 5).

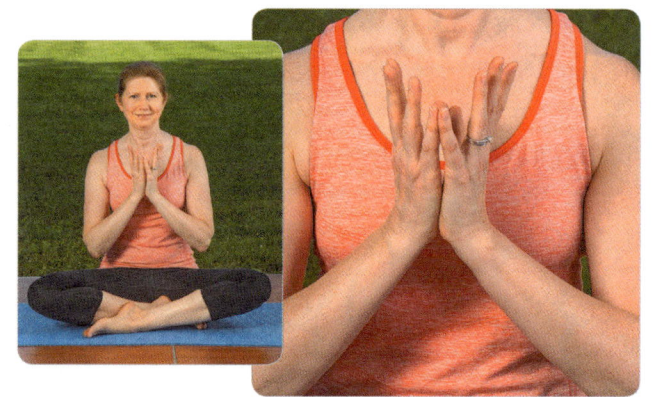

Balance Practice

The Balance Practice helps develop balance on multiple levels. On a physical level, it will help improve your ability to manage the micro-movements that can spell the difference between catching yourself or taking a tumble. On the emotional level, you'll also help balance your mind and emotions. As yoga instructor Laura Malloy, one of the medical editors of this report, says, "It's hard to have a busy mind when you're standing on one foot." But many yoga poses beside the ones in this routine contribute to these skills.

This practice begins with a deep breathing exercise that is unique to this practice. You then perform a number of poses and sequences from the Basic Practice before moving on to some new poses that are specifically aimed at honing your balance. You will continue to alternate various poses from the Basic Practice with new ones from the Balance Practice, until you have done all the poses from the Basic Practice, interspersed with new ones. We do not repeat the instructions for each of the exercises from the Basic Practice, so it helps to have learned them first.

You'll finish the routine with some relaxation and meditation. The complete routine will take about 45 to 60 minutes.

➤ Alternate-nostril breath

Sit comfortably with your spine elongated. Bend your right index and middle fingers downward toward the palm of your hand. Using your thumb, gently close your right nostril and inhale through your left nostril. Bring your ring finger to gently close your left nostril and exhale out of your right nostril. Inhale through your right nostril and close it with your thumb. Exhale through your left nostril. Continue in this way, alternating nostrils for the exhalation. Close your eyes if you like. Breathe slowly. Repeat 10 or more times, ending by exhaling through the left nostril. (For a video demonstration, go to www.health.harvard.edu/alternate-nostril-breath.)

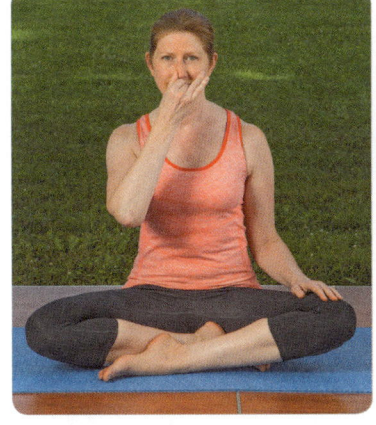
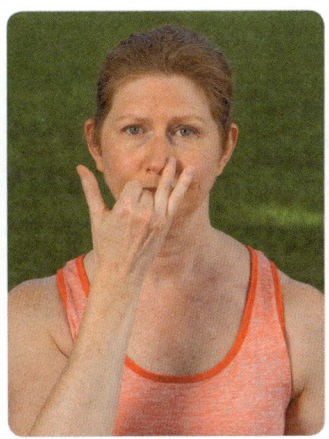
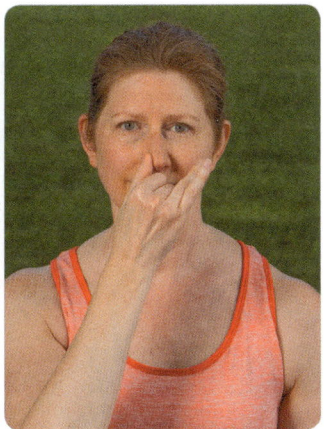

Balance Practice

➤ From the Basic Practice

- Ten churnings (right ankle circles, left ankle circles, head circles, shoulder circles, wrist circles, side stretches, twists, hip circles, knee circles, spine ripples)
- Mountain pose (hold 3 to 6 breaths)
- Half sun salutation (3 times)
- Sun salutation (both sides; see the photo sequence below for a reminder)
- Tree pose (right foot raised)

Sun salutation

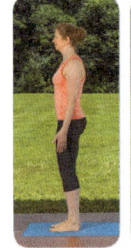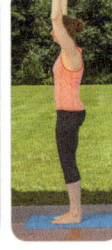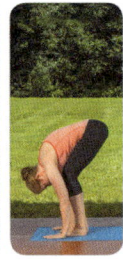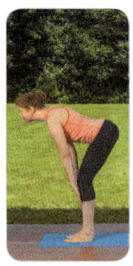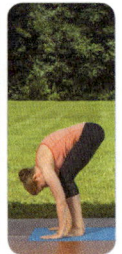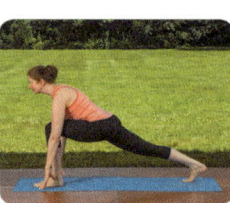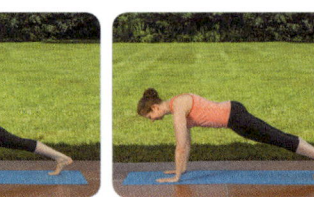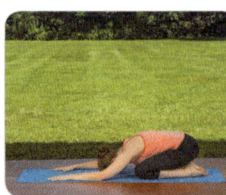

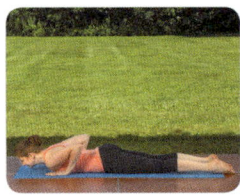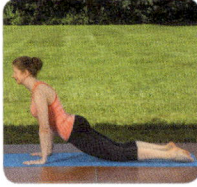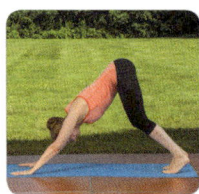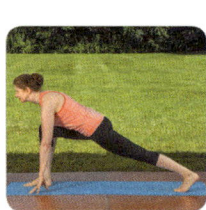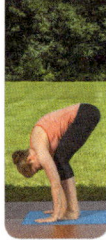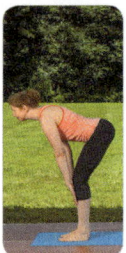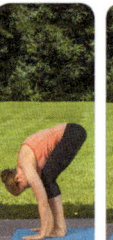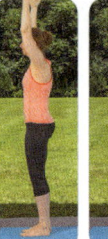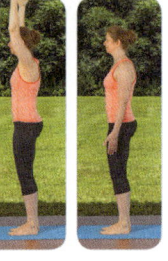

➤ Leg extension balance

Starting position: Mountain pose.

Movement: Raise your right foot in front of you, a few inches off the floor, leg extended and toes pointed. Balancing on your left leg, bend your right knee and bring your left foot in, flexing the foot. Extend and flex three times, with no hold in between. Lower your leg.

Where you'll feel it: Entire body

Reps: 3

Tips and techniques:
- Focus on a stationary spot in front of you to help you balance.
- Drop your tailbone to avoid arching or rounding your back.
- Keep your shoulders relaxed and down, away from your ears.
- Engage your abdominal muscles to stand tall and support your back.
- Keep a slight bend in your standing knee.

Make it easier: Hold on to the back of chair or other sturdy object.

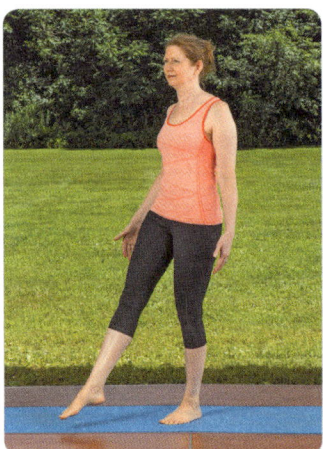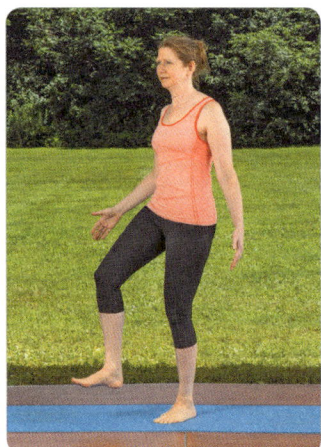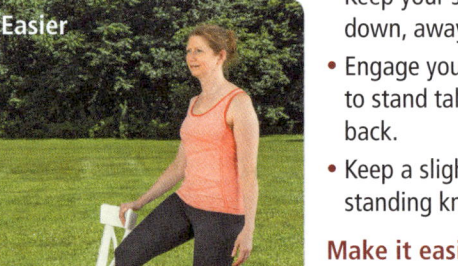

Easier

Balance Practice

➤ Crane

Starting position: Stand tall with your feet slightly apart and your arms out to your sides at shoulder height, elbows bent.

Movement: Balancing on your left leg, raise your right knee to hip height with your foot gently flexed. Hold.

Where you'll feel it: Entire body

Hold: 3 to 6 slow, easy breaths

Reps: 1

Tips and techniques:
- Focus on a stationary spot in front of you to help you balance.
- Drop your tailbone to avoid arching or rounding your back.
- Keep your shoulders relaxed and down, away from your ears.
- Engage your abdominal muscles to stand tall and support your back.

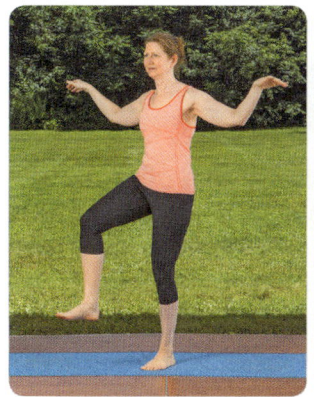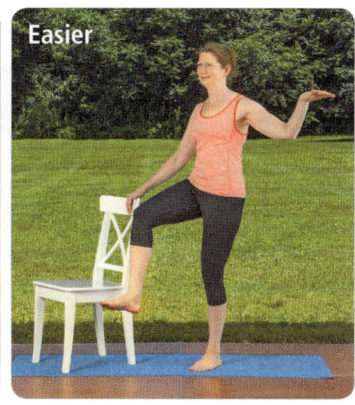

- Keep a slight bend in your standing knee.

Make it easier: Hold on to the back of chair or other sturdy object.

➤ Warrior III

Starting position: Stand tall with your right foot slightly behind you with just your toes on the floor, hands on your hips.

Movement: Keeping a slight bend in your left knee, raise your right foot off the floor behind you as you slowly tip your upper body forward until your right leg and torso are parallel to the floor. When you are stable, extend your arms out to your sides. Hold. Return to starting position.

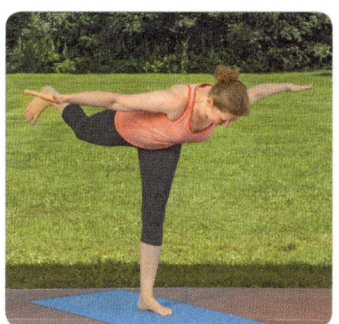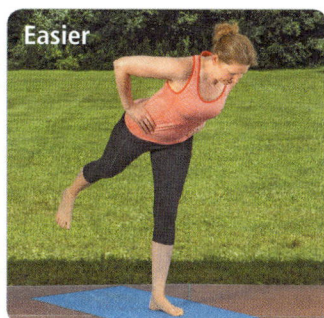

Where you'll feel it: Entire body

Hold: 3 to 6 slow, easy breaths

Reps: 1

Tips and techniques:
- Keep a slight bend in your standing knee.
- Keep your shoulders relaxed, away from your ears.
- Keep your head in line with your spine and look at the floor.
- Keep your shoulders and hips squared and facing the floor.
- Engage your abdominal muscles to support your back.
- Flex your raised foot.

Make it easier: Raise your leg behind you and tip forward only as far as you can comfortably balance with good form. Keep your hands on your hips.

➤ From the Basic Practice

- Warrior II (right foot back)
- Reverse warrior (right foot back)
- Side angle (right foot back)
- Triangle pose (right foot back)
- Mountain pose
- Tree pose (left foot raised)

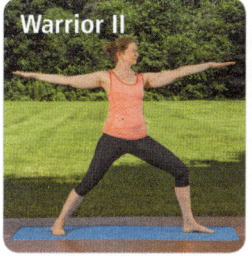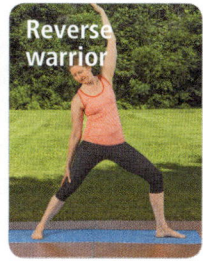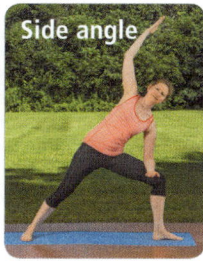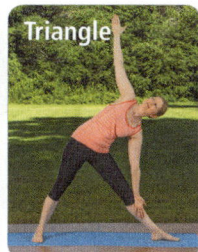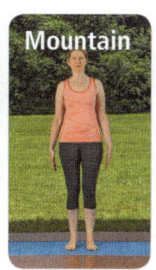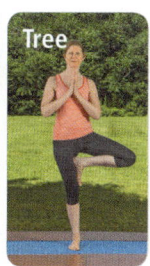

www.health.harvard.edu   Intermediate Yoga   **35**

Balance Practice

➤ Repeat the new moves on the other side
- Leg extension balance (left leg raised)
- Crane (left foot raised)
- Warrior III (left foot raised)

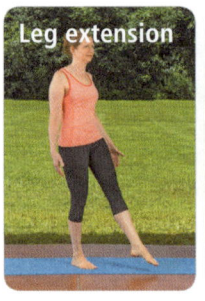
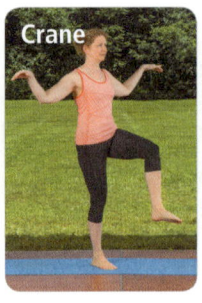
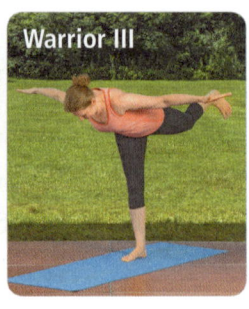

➤ From the Basic Practice
- Warrior II (left foot back)
- Reverse warrior (left foot back)
- Side angle (left foot back)
- Triangle pose (left foot back)
- Mountain pose
- Half sun salutation with downward-facing dog

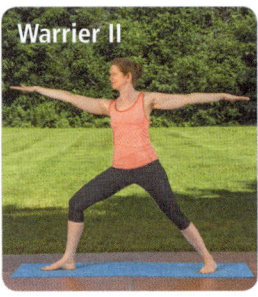
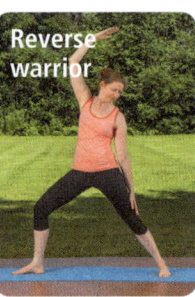
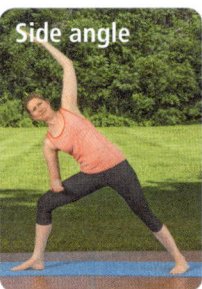
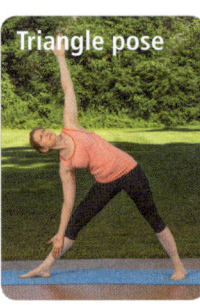
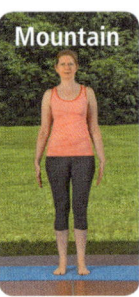

➤ Gate pose

Starting position: Kneel with your arms relaxed at your sides.

Movement: Extend your right leg out to the side with your heel on the floor, toes and knee pointing up toward the ceiling. Inhale and raise your left arm overhead. Exhale and lean toward the right, letting your right hand slide down your leg. Gaze up at your left hand. Hold. Return to the starting position, then repeat with your left leg extended. This completes one rep.

Where you'll feel it: Side of torso

Hold: 3 to 6 slow, easy breaths

Reps: 1

Tips and techniques:
- Place a folded blanket or towel under your knees if needed.
- Keep the foot of your extended leg in line with your bent knee.
- Keep your chest open and facing forward.
- Keep your torso over your extended leg, not leaning forward or backward.

Make it easier: Place your toes down on the floor. Don't bend as far. Gaze straight ahead instead of upward.

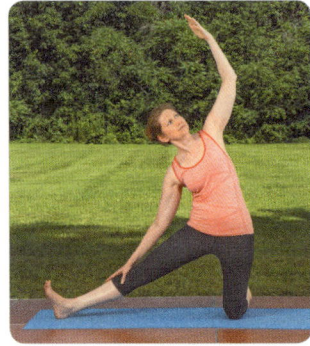
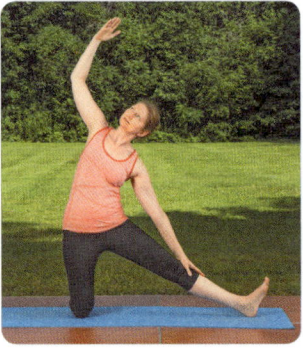
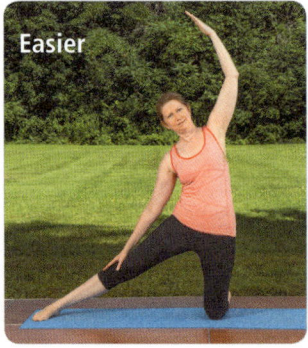

Balance Practice

▸ Extended table

Starting position: Kneel on all fours, knees hip-width apart (tabletop position). Align your shoulders over your wrists and your hips over your knees. Keep your head and spine in neutral alignment.

Movement: Extend your right leg off the floor behind you while reaching your left arm out in front of you. Try to raise your extended leg and arm high enough that they are parallel to the floor. Hold. Return to the starting position, then repeat with your left leg and right arm. This completes one rep.

Where you'll feel it: Arm, shoulder, back, buttocks, leg

Hold: 3 to 6 slow, easy breaths

Reps: 1

Tips and techniques:
- Keep your shoulders and hips level to maintain alignment throughout.
- Keep your head and spine neutral.
- Gaze down at the floor under your nose.
- Engage your abdominal muscles to support your back.
- Think of pulling your hand and leg in opposite directions, lengthening your torso.
- Flex your raised foot.

Make it easier: Lift one arm only and hold, then lift one leg only and hold. Repeat with the opposite arm and leg.

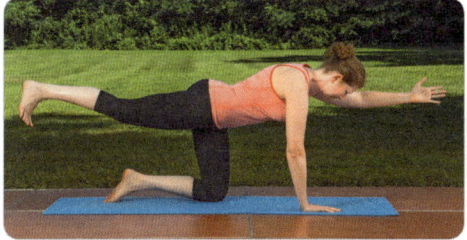 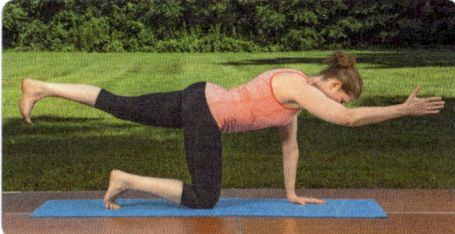 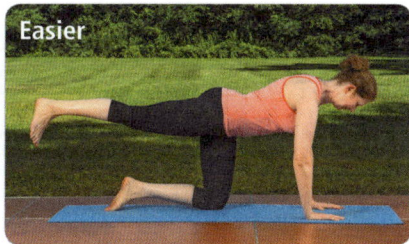

▸ From the Basic Practice

- Seated spinal twist (both sides)
- Bridge pose
- Knees-to-chest
- Wide knee circles (both directions)
- Happy baby pose
- Lying spinal twist (both sides)
- Corpse pose

Finish with the basic breathing meditation (page 27), using the enlightenment mudra (below).

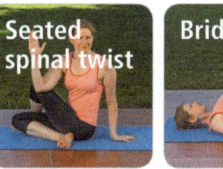 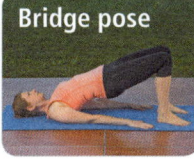 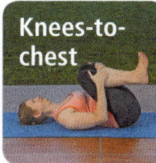 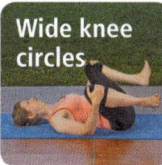 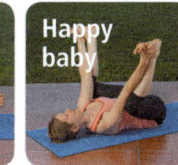 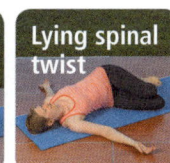 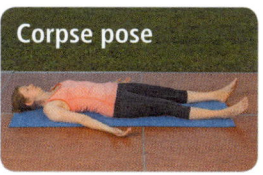

Enlightenment mudra

Start by folding your hands with your fingers interlaced but your palms apart. Your hands should be in front of your chest. Extend both index fingers and press your fingertips together. Do the same with your thumbs, positioning them at a right angle to your other fingers.

The enlightenment mudra has been compared to a lightning rod, but instead of attracting an electrical charge, your index fingers (pointing out) and thumbs (pointing toward you) help you draw hope and inspiration from the universe and direct them toward yourself. The interlaced middle, ring, and little fingers symbolize unity and connectedness.

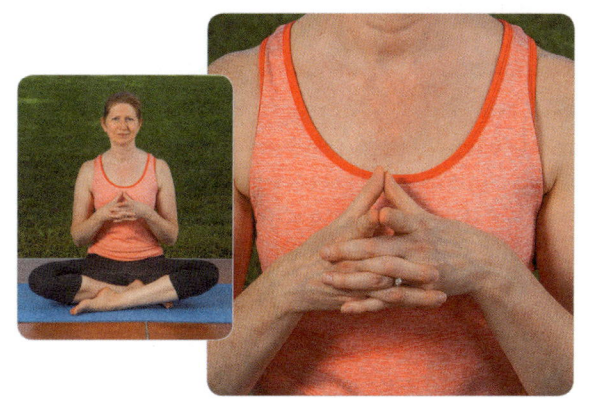

Intermediate Yoga

Strengthening Practice

The Strengthening Practice targets your entire body, helping you build a strong lower body, core, and upper body. As you advance in your practice, try to think of strength in more than just physical terms. While you do this practice, hold the intention in your mind of developing mental and psychological strength to help support yourself and others to overcome life's challenges.

This practice begins with a deep breathing exercise that is unique to this practice. You then perform a number of poses and sequences from the Basic Practice before moving on to some new poses that are specifically aimed at increasing your strength. You will continue to alternate various poses from the Basic Practice with new ones from the Strengthening Practice, until you have done all the poses from the Basic Practice, interspersed with new ones. We do not repeat the instructions for each of the exercises from the Basic Practice, so it helps to have learned them first.

You'll finish the routine with some relaxation and meditation. The complete routine will take about 45 to 60 minutes.

➤ Bellows breath

Sit comfortably with your spine long. As you inhale through your nose, raise your arms straight overhead, with your hands open, palms facing forward. Exhale vigorously through your nose and quickly draw your hands into fists at your shoulders. Close your eyes if you like. Repeat at a steady pace for 10 rounds. You can do up to 3 repetitions of this. (For a video demonstration, go to www.health.harvard.edu/bellows-breath.) Avoid this breath is you are pregnant or you have a heart or respiratory problem.

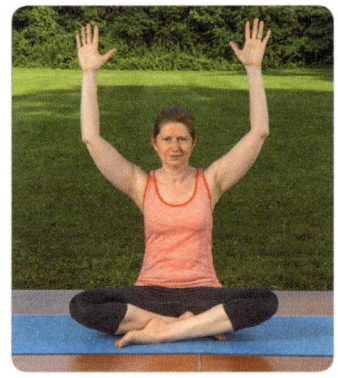
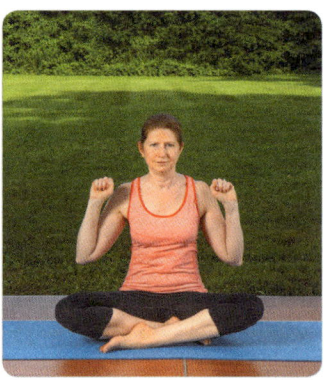

➤ From the Basic Practice

- Ten churnings (right ankle circles, left ankle circles, head circles, shoulder circles, wrist circles, side stretches, twists, hip circles, knee circles, spine ripples)
- Mountain pose
- Half sun salutation (3 times)
- Sun salutation (both sides)

➤ Chair pose

Starting position: Mountain pose.

Movement: As you inhale, raise your arms overhead. As you exhale, bend your hips and knees and lower yourself into a squat position, keeping your back neutral. Hold. Inhale as you stand back up. Lower your arms as you exhale.

Where you'll feel it: Buttocks, hips, legs, shoulders

Hold: 3 to 6 slow, easy breaths

Reps: 1

Tips and techniques:
- Engage your abdominal muscles to support your back.
- Keep your knees no farther forward than your toes as you sit back.

Make it easier: Squat only halfway. Raise your arms to chest height only, or keep your hands on your hips.

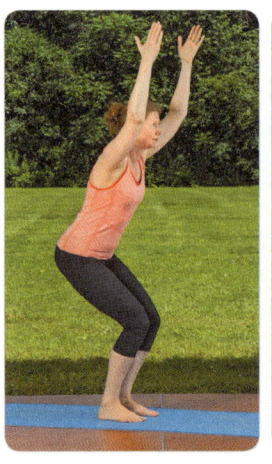
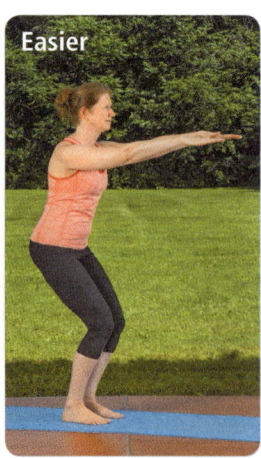

➤ From the Basic Practice

- Tree pose (right foot raised)

➤ Warrior I

Starting position: Stand tall with your feet about hip-width apart, arms relaxed down at your sides. Inhale.

Movement: On an exhale, step back with your right foot, so that your right foot is angled inward and your left foot pointing forward, and bend your left knee, lowering into a lunge. As you inhale, raise your arms up overhead. Hold.

Where you'll feel it: Legs, buttocks, back, shoulders, arms

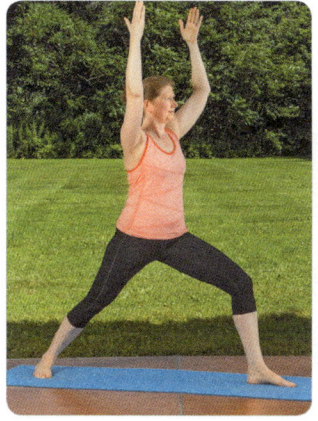 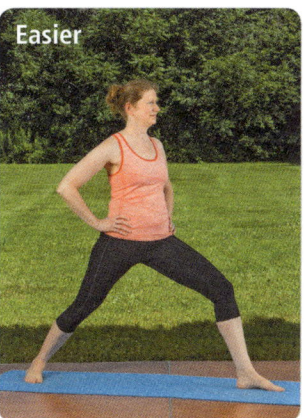

Hold: 3 to 6 slow, easy breaths

Reps: 1

Tips and techniques:
- Keep your front knee over your ankle.
- Keep your tailbone tucked and your back straight.
- Keep your hips and shoulders squared and facing forward.

Make it easier: Place your hands on your hips. Don't lower as far down into the lunge.

➤ From the Basic Practice

- Warrior II (right foot back)
- Reverse warrior (right foot back)
- Side angle (right foot back)
- Triangle pose (right foot back)
- Mountain pose
- Tree pose (left foot raised)
- Warrior I (left foot back; from the Strengthening Practice, above)

- Warrior II (left foot back)
- Reverse warrior (left foot back)
- Side angle (left foot back)
- Triangle pose (left foot back)
- Mountain pose
- Half sun salutation with downward-facing dog

➤ Locust

Starting position: Lie facedown on the floor with your arms by your sides, palms down, your legs extended, and toes pointed.

Movement: Simultaneously lift your head, chest, arms, and legs off the floor as high as is comfortable, supporting yourself on your abdomen and pelvis. Release on an exhale, slowly lowering your body back down to the floor. Relax in child's pose for 3 to 6 breaths before moving on to the next move.

Where you'll feel it: Back

Hold: 3 to 6 slow, easy breaths

Reps: 1

Tips and techniques:
- Tighten your inner thighs to lift your legs.
- Don't bend your knees.
- Keep your gaze down.
- Keep your shoulders down, away from your ears.

Make it easier: Don't lift as high. Or, lift your upper body only, and then lift your lower body only.

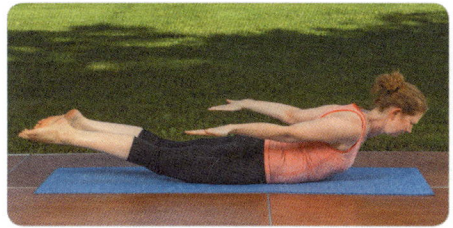 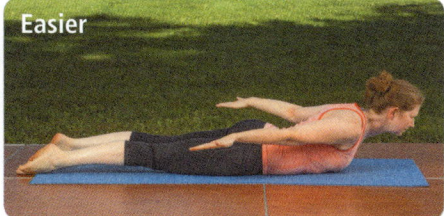 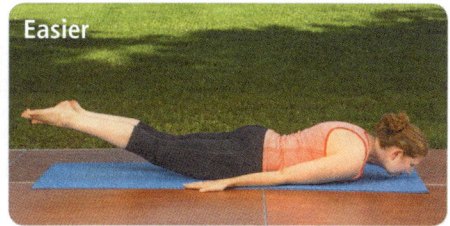

Strengthening Practice

➤ Dolphin

Starting position: Kneel on all fours with your knees under your hips, and then lower onto your elbows and forearms. Bring the palms of your hands together, and tuck your toes.

Movement: Straighten your legs, lifting your hips toward the ceiling, so you form an inverted V with your body.

Where you'll feel it: Back, arms, legs

Hold: 3 to 6 slow, easy breaths

Reps: 1

Tips and techniques:
- Draw your shoulder blades down your back, away from your ears.
- Relax your neck; keep your ears in line with your upper arms.
- Keep the weight on your elbows and forearms.
- Keep a gentle bend in your knees.

Make it easier: Don't raise your knees as high off the floor.

If you have back problems or glaucoma, check with your doctor before doing this move.

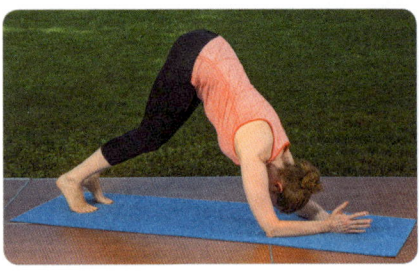
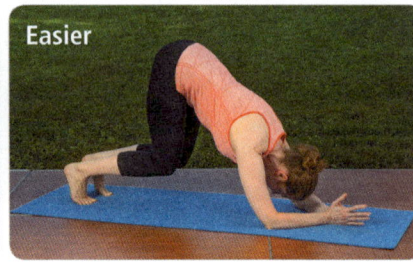

➤ Half boat pose

Starting position: Sit on the floor with your knees bent and feet flat on the floor. Hold on to the underside of your thighs.

Movement: Lift your feet off the floor so your shins are parallel to the floor to form a V with your upper body and thighs. Raise your arms out to your sides with your palms up. Hold.

Where you'll feel it: Abdomen

Hold: 3 to 6 slow, easy breaths

Reps: 1

Tips and techniques:
- Don't round your back.
- Draw your shoulder blades down your back, away from your ears.
- Don't let your chin jut forward; keep it slightly tucked.
- Keep your chest lifted.

Make it easier: Continue to hold on to the back of your thighs, and don't lift your feet as high. You can even keep your toes touching the floor.

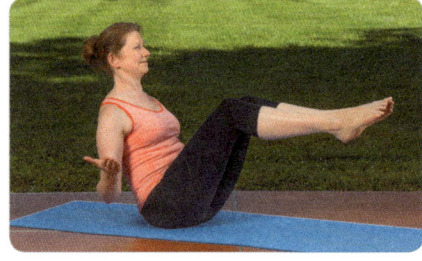
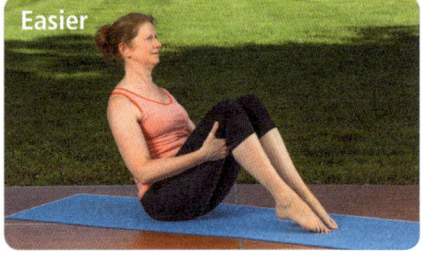

➤ From the Basic Practice

- Seated spinal twist (both sides)
- Bridge pose
- Knees-to-chest
- Wide knee circles (both directions)
- Happy baby pose
- Lying spinal twist (both sides)
- Corpse pose

Finish with the basic breathing meditation (page 27), using the overcoming mudra (below).

Overcoming mudra

With your left palm facing away from you and your right palm facing toward you, bend and grasp your fingers. Draw your elbows out to the sides and hold your hands in front of your chest.

While holding this mudra, you're doing an isometric contraction, which can build physical strength. But the position is also intended to build internal strengths like perseverance, resilience, and courage. It can be a morale booster when you're feeling down. It pairs well with ujjayi breath (see page 44) in addition to the basic breathing meditation. ▼

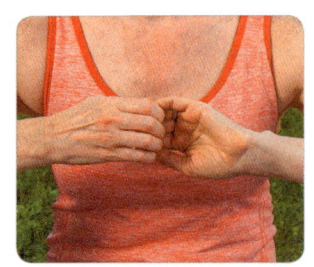

Energizing Practice

Get ready for a jolt of vitality as you embark on this practice. The vigorous breathing will bring more oxygen to your body and brain for both physical and mental energy, while expanding your chest in the camel pose (page 42) will help lift your mood. You'll be ready to embrace each new day with more vigor and have the stamina to power through, staying sharp and focused until night.

This practice begins with a deep breathing exercise that is unique to this practice. You then perform a number of poses and sequences from the Basic Practice before moving on to some new poses that are specifically aimed at increasing your energy. You will continue to alternate various poses from the Basic Practice with new ones from the Energizing Practice, until you have done all the poses from the Basic Practice, interspersed with new ones. We do not repeat the instructions for each of the exercises from the Basic Practice, so it helps to have learned them first.

You'll finish the routine with some relaxation and meditation. The complete routine will take about 45 to 60 minutes.

➤ Breath of joy

Stand with your feet wider than hip-width apart, with your arms down at your sides. Take a quick, short inhale through the nose as you swing your arms up into each of these three positions—in front at shoulder height, straight out to the sides, and up overhead. Let your arms swing down to your sides before moving to each new position. End by exhaling through the mouth with a short, sharp "ha" as you hinge forward at your hips, swinging your arms behind you. Straighten up again, and repeat this sequence 3 to 6 times. At the end, shake out your arms and legs to release any tension. (For a video demonstration, go to www.health.harvard.edu/breath-of-joy.)

If you haven't warmed up, hinge slowly at first until your muscles loosen up. If it is not recommended for you to hinge forward, simply bring your arms down to your sides instead of bending forward on the last move.

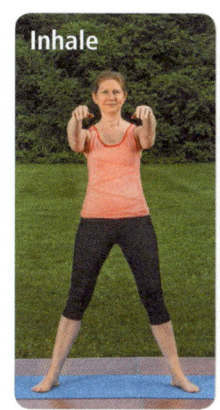
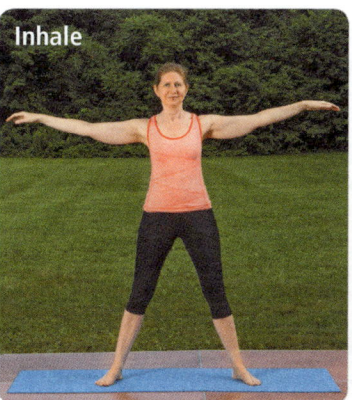
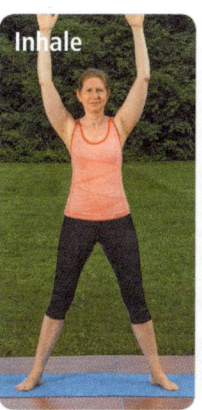
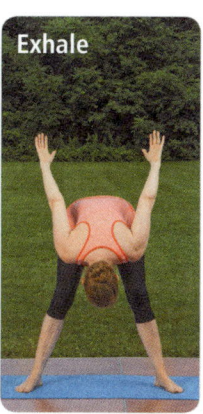

➤ From the Basic Practice

- Ten churnings (right ankle circles, left ankle circles, head circles, shoulder circles, wrist circles, side stretches, twists, hip circles, knee circles, spine ripples)
- Mountain pose
- Half sun salutation (3 times)
- Sun salutation (both sides)
- Tree pose (right foot raised)
- Warrior II (right foot back)
- Reverse warrior (right foot back)
- Side angle (right foot back)
- Triangle pose (right foot back)
- Mountain pose
- Tree pose (left foot raised)
- Warrior II (left foot back)
- Reverse warrior (left foot back)
- Side angle (left foot back)
- Triangle pose (left foot back)

Energizing Practice

➤ Five-pointed star into goddess with lion's breath

Starting position: Stand tall with your feet wider than shoulder-width apart, toes angled slightly out. Inhale and extend your arms out to your sides at shoulder height (five-pointed star).

Movement: Inhale through your nose. Then exhale though your mouth, sticking your tongue out, with a long "haaaa" (the lion's breath). As you perform the lion's breath, bend your knees and your arms, lowering into a squat with your arms in a goalpost position (goddess pose; for a demonstration, go to www.health.harvard.edu/lions-breath). Return to the starting position.

Where you'll feel it: Back, buttocks, legs, upper arms

Reps: 3

Tips and techniques:
- When your arms are extended, reach to the sides.
- Keep your shoulders relaxed and down, away from your ears.
- Keep your weight evenly balanced between your feet.
- Engage your abdominal muscles to support your back.

Make it easier: Don't lower so far into the squat.

If you have back problems or osteoporosis, check with your doctor before doing this move.

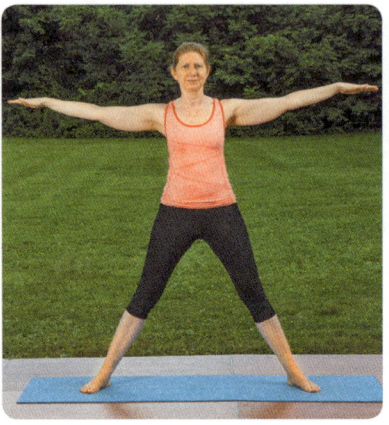
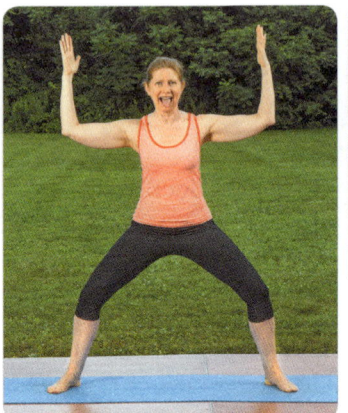
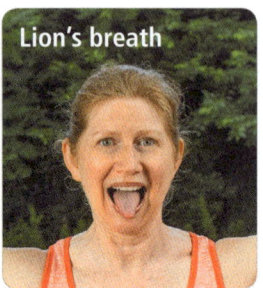
Lion's breath

➤ From the Basic Practice
- Mountain pose
- Half sun salutation with downward-facing dog

➤ Camel

Starting position: Kneel with your toes tucked under and your arms relaxed at your sides.

Movement: Open up your chest and reach with your right hand back to your right heel. Then reach with your left hand back to your left heel. Keep your gaze upward and press your hips forward. Hold. Slowly return to the starting position.

Where you'll feel it: Chest, shoulders

Hold: 3 to 6 slow, easy breaths

Reps: 1

Tips and techniques:
- Place a folded blanket or towel under your knees if needed.
- Keep your tailbone down to protect your lower back.
- Think about lengthening your spine as you arch back.
- Don't let your chin jut forward; keep it slightly tucked.
- Keep your thighs as vertical as possible, not leaning backward.

Make it easier: Place your hands on the small of your back instead of your heels.

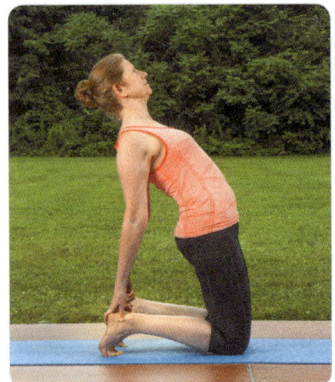
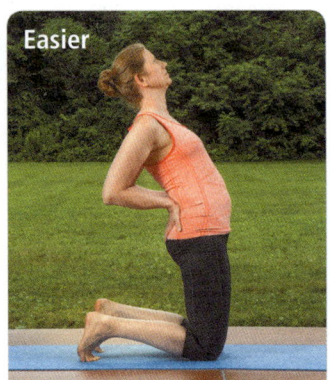
Easier

Energizing Practice

➤ Reverse plank

Starting position: Sit up straight on the floor with your legs together and extended in front of you, toes pointed. Place your hands on the floor behind you, fingers pointing toward you.

Movement: On an inhale, press into your hands and your heels and lift your buttocks and legs off the floor until your body is in line from shoulders to hips to feet. Hold.

Where you'll feel it: Entire body

Hold: 3 to 6 slow, easy breaths

Reps: 1

Tips and techniques:
- Don't lock your elbows.
- Draw your shoulder blades down your back, away from your ears.
- Point your toes.
- Don't drop your head backward.

Make it easier: Put your elbows down, and lift your buttocks and legs just a few inches off the floor.

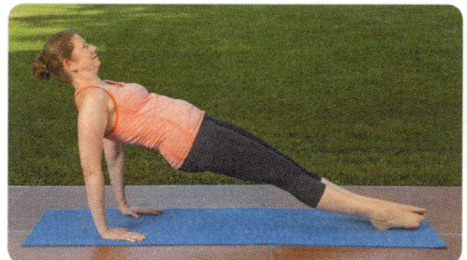
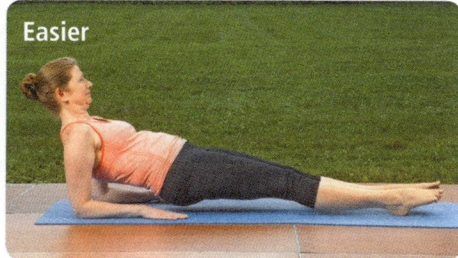

Easier

➤ From the Basic Practice

- Seated spinal twist (both sides)
- Bridge pose
- Knees-to-chest
- Wide knee circles (both directions)
- Happy baby pose
- Lying spinal twist (both sides)
- Corpse pose

Finish with the basic breathing meditation (page 27), using the energy mudra (below).

Energy mudra

Press the tip of your thumb to your middle and ring fingers on each hand. Extend your index and little fingers so they are straight. Rest your hands in your lap or on your legs with your palms facing up.

Feel the energy coming in through your fingertips. With each inhale, imagine breathing in positive energy and thoughts like "I am healthy," "I am strong." On each exhale, release any negative energy or thoughts. You can also pair this mudra with ujjayi breath (see page 44). ♥

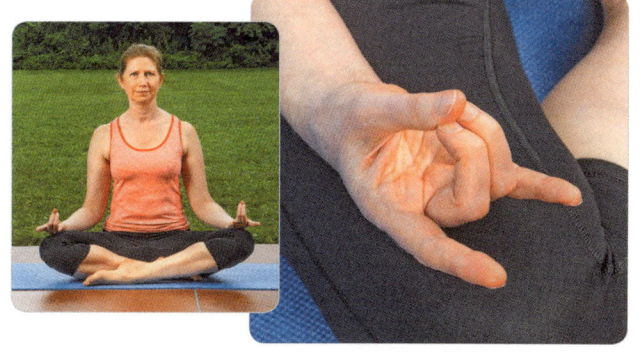

Calming Practice

You might think of the Calming Practice as something to do in the evening, when your work for the day is finished, but this routine can be done any time of day. For example, when you're anxious or worked up over something, this practice can center and relax you.

This practice begins with a deep breathing exercise that is unique to this practice. You then perform a number of poses and sequences from the Basic Practice before moving on to some new poses that are specifically aimed at calming you down. You will continue to alternate various poses from the Basic Practice with new ones from the Calming Practice, until you have done all the poses from the Basic Practice, interspersed with new ones. We do not repeat the instructions for each of the exercises from the Basic Practice, so it helps to have learned them first.

You'll finish the routine with some relaxation and meditation. The complete routine will take about 45 to 60 minutes.

➤ Ujjayi breath

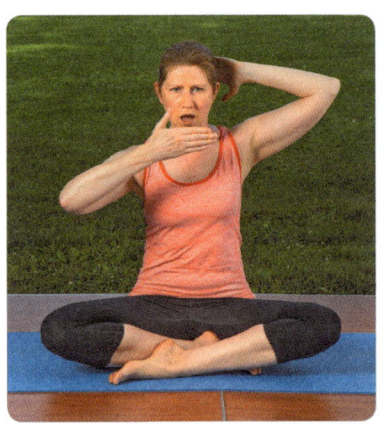

Sit comfortably with your spine elongated. Hold one palm a few inches in front of your mouth and one palm an inch or two behind your head. Inhale and exhale through your mouth. As you exhale, make a long "haaaa" sound, letting your breath warm the palm of your front hand, as if it were a mirror you were trying to fog. Imagine the hand behind you is also a mirror and make a long "haaaa" sound as you inhale as if you could fog that as well. Do this 3 times and then place your hands down in your lap. Slightly tuck your chin to your chest. Inhale and exhale though your nose while gently constricting the muscles in the back of your throat to make the same "ha" sound that you made through your mouth. The sound will be like that of ocean waves. Close your eyes if you like. Breathe slowly. Repeat 6 to 10 times. (For a video demonstration, go to www.health.harvard.edu/ujjayi-breath.)

➤ From the Basic Practice

- Ten churnings (right ankle circles, left ankle circles, head circles, shoulder circles, wrist circles, side stretches, twists, hip circles, knee circles, spine ripples)
- Mountain pose
- Half sun salutation (3 times)
- Sun salutation (both sides)
- Tree pose (right foot raised)
- Warrior II (right foot back)
- Reverse warrior (right foot back)
- Side angle (right foot back)
- Triangle pose (right foot back)
- Mountain pose
- Tree pose (left foot raised)
- Warrior II (left foot back)
- Reverse warrior (left foot back)
- Side angle (left foot back)
- Triangle pose (left foot back)
- Mountain pose
- Half sun salutation

Calming Practice

➤ Ragdoll

Starting position: Forward fold.

Movement: Shift your feet a little wider apart. Grasp each elbow with the opposite hand and bend your knees so your chest is closer to your thighs. Gently sway side to side as you breathe deeply.

Where you'll feel it: Shoulders, back, backs of thighs

Reps: 6 sways to each side

Tips and techniques:
- Keep your shoulders relaxed and down, away from your ears.
- Let your head relax and hang freely.
- Tighten your abdominal muscles to support your back.

Make it easier: Place your hands on the seat of a chair.

If you have back problems, glaucoma, or osteoporosis, check with your doctor before doing this move.

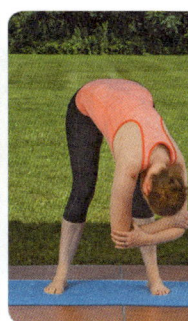 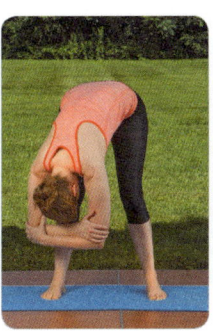 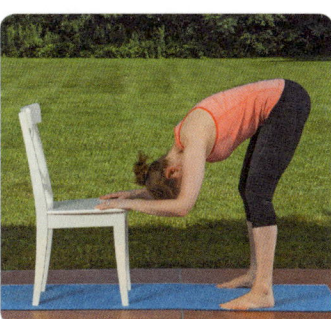

➤ From the Basic Practice

- Downward-facing dog

➤ Cat-cow

Starting position: Get down on all fours with your hands directly beneath your shoulders and your knees beneath your hips (tabletop position). Keep your back flat.

Movement: As you inhale, lift your tailbone and chest toward the ceiling like a cow. As you exhale, round your back, tucking your tailbone under and bringing your chin toward your chest like a cat. That's one rep. Continue moving with your breath; do not hold.

Where you'll feel it: Chest, back, backs of thighs

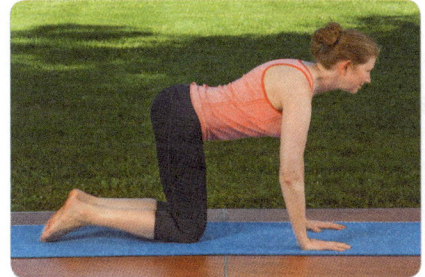 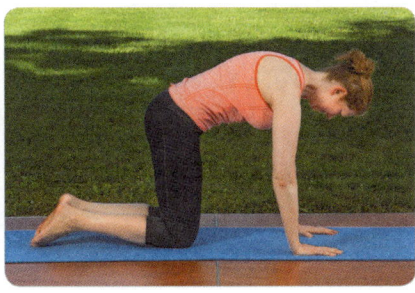

Reps: 3 to 6

Tips and techniques:
- Keep the movement slow and controlled.
- Don't overarch your back.

Make it easier: Don't arch the spine as much in cat. Don't raise the chest as much in cow.

If you have back problems or osteoporosis, check with your doctor before doing this move.

Calming Practice

➤ Thread the needle

Starting position: Remain on all fours with your hands directly beneath your shoulders and your knees beneath your hips (tabletop position).

Movement: As you inhale, raise your right arm out to the side, palm down. As you exhale, bring your right arm under your body and slide it behind your left arm, palm up, as you lower your right shoulder and temple to the floor. Keep your hips lifted. Hold. Return to starting position and repeat with your left arm.

Where you'll feel it: Shoulders, upper back

Hold: 3 to 6 slow, easy breaths

Reps: 1

Tips and techniques:
- Keep your thighs vertical, not leaning to the side.
- Don't sit back on your heels.

Make it easier: Keep your head and shoulder off the floor.

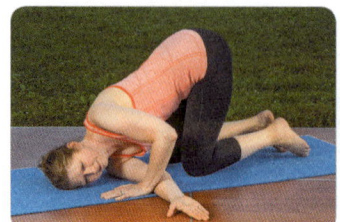 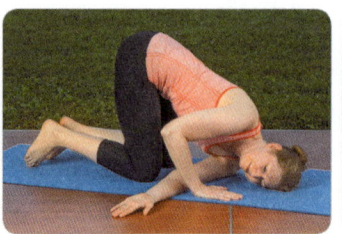 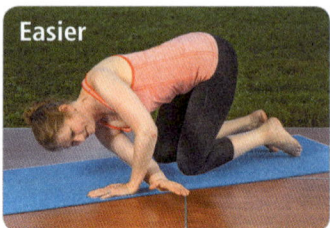

➤ From the Basic Practice

- Child's pose
- Seated spinal twist (both sides)
- Bridge pose
- Knees-to-chest
- Wide knee circles (both directions)
- Happy baby pose
- Lying spinal twist (both sides)

➤ Reclined bound angle

Starting position: Lie faceup on the floor with your arms and legs comfortably apart and your palms facing up.

Movement: Bring the soles of your feet together, letting your knees fall out to the sides. Hold.

Where you'll feel it: Entire body

Hold: 3 to 6 slow, easy breaths

Reps: 1

Tips and techniques:
- Keep your head neutral, not tilted back or tucked toward your chin.
- Try not to arch your back.

Make it easier: Place rolled-up towels, blankets, or blocks under your knees or thighs, if needed. Or bring the feet farther away from your buttocks.

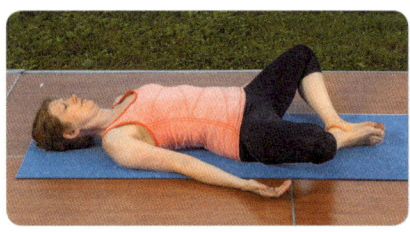 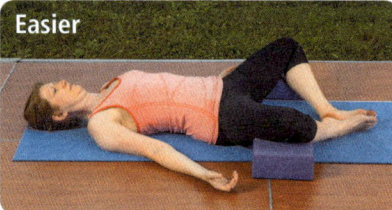

➤ From the Basic Practice

- Corpse pose

Finish with the basic breathing meditation (page 27), using the meditation mudra (below).

Meditation mudra

Rest one hand on top of the other with your palms up. Touch the tips of your thumbs together to form a circle with your hands. Rest your hands in your lap or hold them in front of your navel.

This mudra may look familiar since the Buddha is often depicted in meditation with his hands held like this. It's commonly used for meditation and breathing exercises as a way for you to center yourself. It's a good idea to switch hands partway through or each time you do it, so the opposite hand is on top. The change from what is natural can make you more aware of your body. ▼

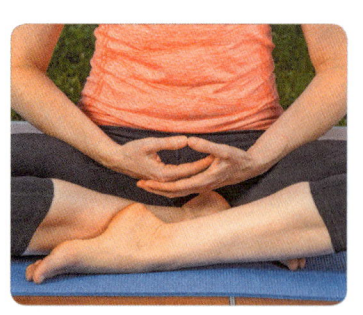

SPECIAL SECTION

Expand your practice—finding the right class

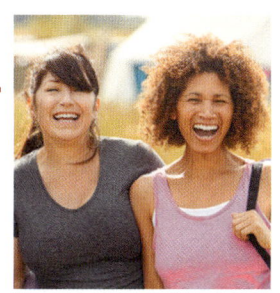

The program presented in this report is a good foundation for a yoga practice. But at some point, you may want to engage in additional practices with greater diversity, depth, and challenge. In-person group classes, online classes, and apps can all provide new routines. Two popular yoga apps are Yoga Studio and Daily Yoga. You can also find hundreds of yoga workouts online. Yoga teacher Adriene Mishler offers free videos on her website Yoga with Adriene (www.yogawithadriene.com). You might also want to check out subscription-based sites like Yoga International.com and Glo.com for online and livestreamed classes. (See "Resources," page 53, for more information.)

Finding an appropriate in-person or virtual class and instructor will take some effort and care. The guidelines below focus on in-person classes, but you can apply many of them when evaluating virtual programs, too.

Selecting a type of yoga

Your first step in searching for a class is simply to choose a style of yoga that you would like to practice. No style is better than another—it's all about finding what's right for you, given your fitness level and goals. Some styles of yoga are vigorous, while others are slow-paced and gentle. Some use props to help you with poses. Some are done mainly lying down. Yoga's popularity has spurred the proliferation of styles, along with some interesting variations (see "More types of yoga," page 49). The program outlined in this report is largely a Kripalu style.

Here is an overview of the most common styles, with an eye to the main focus, intent, and unique characteristics of each one. The good news is that with most styles of yoga, you'll release tension and relax. Additional benefits depend upon the type of yoga you select.

Hatha yoga

Hatha is a generic term, referring to the practice of physical postures. As such, most styles of yoga practiced in the West are technically Hatha. In the United States, however, gyms and community centers often use the term Hatha to describe a basic or gentle yoga. Hatha classes combine breathing exercises with simple postures done at a slow pace and often held for a few breaths. Most classes include some relaxation at the end. Hatha is meant to prepare the practitioner for meditation. It is also helpful for stress reduction. In a study published in the journal *Complementary Therapies in Medicine*, just one 30-minute Hatha class helped participants respond to and recover from stress better than watching TV.

Integral yoga

While gentle and noncompetitive, integral yoga is a comprehensive

www.health.harvard.edu   Intermediate Yoga   47

SPECIAL SECTION | Expand your practice—finding the right class

practice that includes chanting, postures, deep relaxation, breathing practices, and meditations. This type of yoga seeks to integrate the mind, body, and spirit and give students tools to live peaceful, healthy, joyful, useful lives. The yoga used in Dr. Dean Ornish's heart disease reversal program is rooted in integral yoga.

Iyengar yoga

This style was developed by the renowned yogi B.K.S. Iyengar, who helped popularize yoga in India and abroad in the 20th century. It emphasizes proper alignment in order to maximize benefits. Classes often focus on fewer poses, but explore the subtle effects that body position has on a particular posture—for example, turning your foot slightly out instead of straight ahead for a more effective stretch. Yoga blocks, straps, blankets, chairs, or other props are often used in Iyengar classes to allow you to work within a comfortable range of motion. For example, there's no need to touch your toes if that's too much of a stretch for you. Instead, you can simply place your hands on a chair or yoga block at the point that provides a gentle stretch. The attention to proper form makes it a good choice if you have injuries or pain issues. It is also the style of yoga that has been used in many studies of the elderly, breast cancer patients, and people with cardiac problems.

Yin yoga

In ancient Chinese philosophy, yin and yang represent two opposing, yet complementary, forces that pervade the natural world. Yang is masculine, while yin is feminine. Yang is active and hot, while yin is passive and cold. All manner of things can be categorized in this way, including styles of yoga. Yang styles are vigorous, muscle-building approaches like Ashtanga and Vinyasa (see page 50). Yin styles are slower and more contemplative.

The style that actually bears the name yin yoga encourages practitioners to go deeper into poses by holding them longer—for beginners, perhaps a minute, building up to three to five minutes, though some advanced practitioners hold them as long as 20 minutes. Going deeper into poses can help release muscle tension and lengthen connective tissues for greater flexibility and range of motion. Most of the poses are done while sitting or lying down to help muscles fully relax. Sometimes props are used to facilitate the longer holds, but even with them, you may notice deeper, more intense sensations, what some yogis call "comfortable discomfort." That's why breathing is also a primary component of this practice. It gives you something to focus on as you hold difficult or uncomfortable postures, making it a much more meditative style.

Restorative yoga

Relaxation is the primary goal of restorative yoga classes. You do simple poses, most of them while lying down, and rest in each pose for several minutes, some even up to 10 minutes. To make the holding part easier, you use props such as blankets, pillows, or bolsters to support your body so you can

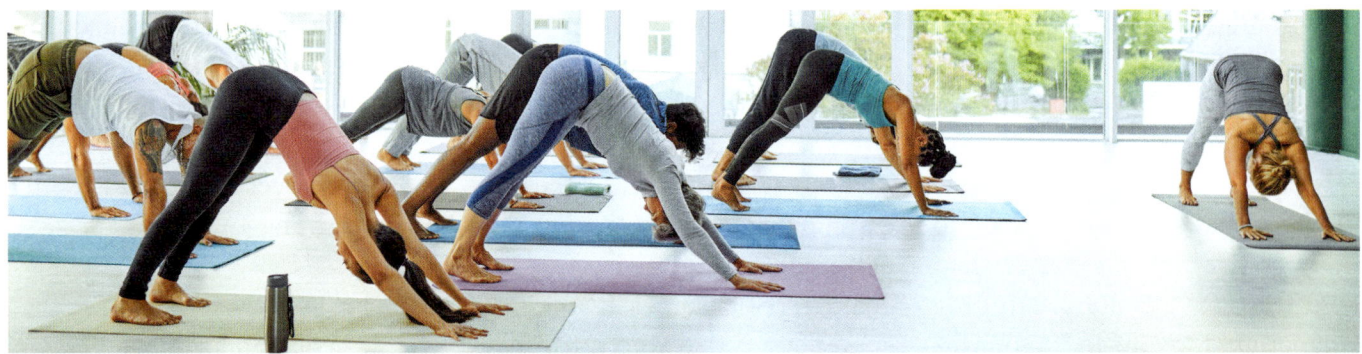

No style of yoga is better than another. It's all about finding what's right for you, given your fitness level, preferences, and goals.

fully relax. You'll also likely be led through a guided meditation. Several studies show that this type of yoga may help people with cancer cope better by reducing fatigue and physical discomfort, improving sleep, and enhancing emotional well-being. It's a great option for the elderly or anyone with physical ailments or restrictions. However, anyone who needs to slow down and release tension can benefit. Restorative yoga is also a great recovery-day activity between harder workouts.

Kripalu yoga

Kripalu yoga, which incorporates all the traditional eight limbs of yoga, is known as the yoga of consciousness. This introspective practice integrates body, mind, and energy with an emphasis on inner psychological and spiritual development. Kripalu means compassion, and you are invited to cultivate compassion for yourself, however you are feeling physically or emotionally in your practice. As you do postures, breathing exercises, meditation, and relaxation techniques, you pay attention to the physical sensations in your body, emotions, and thoughts to increase mind-body awareness and mindfulness. Classes can be physically demanding or extremely gentle, such as chair yoga.

Viniyoga

While most of the other types of yoga can be done in a group setting, Viniyoga involves private instruction and adaptation. With a therapeutic focus, an experienced instructor personalizes the yoga based on a person's health, age, interests, and physical condition, including past and current injuries or limitations. The one-on-one instruction provides more attention to proper alignment than is possible in a group setting. Poses tend to be held for a consistent number of breaths with rest in between. This style may be good for you if you have injuries, physical limitations, or unique needs that may require more modifications; if you want extra personal attention to improve alignment; or if you want a customized practice.

More types of yoga

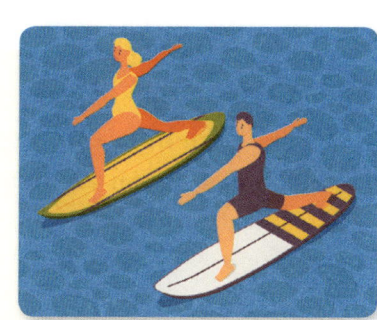

Did you know that there are classes where people do yoga with baby goats, or while wrapped in fabric and suspended in the air? There are also growing numbers of hybrid classes, such as Koga (kickboxing + yoga), Yogilates (yoga + Pilates), and Doga (yoga with your dog). Not all of these meet with approval from purists. But some variations on traditional yoga may be worth considering. Here are some you may come across.

Laughter yoga. This is no joke! Laughter yoga consists of physical exercise, such as clapping, arm and leg movements, and gentle neck and shoulder stretches; relaxation techniques; and simulated smiling and vigorous laughter—although at some point it probably becomes involuntary. Not surprisingly, it's been found to make people feel better and lower levels of the stress hormone cortisol. Even people with serious medical conditions—for example, those awaiting organ transplants or undergoing dialysis—have been shown to benefit, and their nurses have noticed the improvements in them, too. To find a class or for more information, go to the website of Laughter Yoga International at www.laughteryoga.org.

Aqua yoga. As the name implies, this is yoga done in a pool. You don't do moves underwater, but you often use the pool wall as if it's the floor. Yoga is low-impact to begin with, but doing it in water reduces the pressure on your joints even more. That's why it's a good option for people with arthritis, joint replacements, multiple sclerosis, fibromyalgia, or other conditions that make moving difficult or painful. For healthy practitioners, it offers variety and a new experience. Check with pools in your area to find a class.

SUP (stand up paddleboard) yoga. For a real balance challenge, try this popular class that's done on top of water while standing on a paddleboard. It requires more focus and strength because you're not grounded like you are in land-based classes. But the scenery and fresh air can add to its restorative power. Start in calm waters on calm days, since waves and wind increase the challenge. And be prepared to get wet and have fun (you might even get a dose of laughter yoga in this class). Check with paddleboard rental companies to find classes.

SPECIAL SECTION | Expand your practice—finding the right class

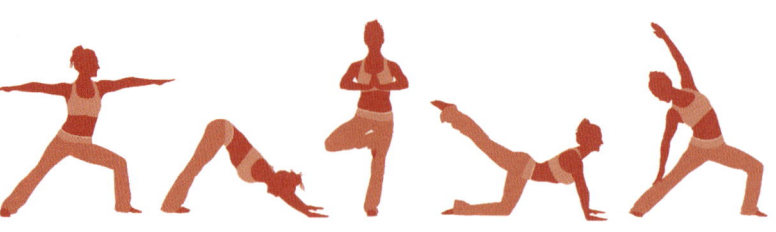

Vinyasa yoga
A Vinyasa practice links movement with breath. Each inhalation and exhalation is matched to a posture or a transition from one posture to the next. The most well-known Vinyasa sequence is the sun salutation (see page 21). Some gentle Vinyasa classes may be called "flow yoga," while more vigorous ones are often called "power yoga." A Vinyasa class may be a good option if you have a hard time sitting still or if you are looking to get some cardio benefits from your practice.

Ashtanga yoga
The goal of this vigorous, athletic practice is to produce internal heat, resulting in sweating and increased circulation. In an Ashtanga class, you flow through a specific series of postures that are synchronized with your breathing. The postures are always the same from class to class, and you use a unique breathing style called ujjayi (see page 44). This type of breathing is characterized by an ocean sound (some people refer to it as a Darth Vader sound), which resonates in the throat and provides a focal point as you practice. The vigorous nature of this style can help you to build stamina and may increase cardio fitness.

Bikram or hot yoga
These styles of yoga are done in rooms that are heated to as much as 105° F. While the heat can help improve flexibility, the high temperature may be dangerous for people with certain medical conditions. If you have diabetes, heart disease, respiratory disease, or a history of heat-related illness, or if you take any medications (some may interfere with your body's ability to regulate heat), check with your doctor before taking a Bikram or hot yoga class. Traditional Bikram classes are 90 minutes long and feature a flowing series of 26 poses that is done twice (the same poses in every class), with breathing exercises in between. Other hot yoga classes usually follow a similar format, but the poses vary.

Jivamukti yoga
This vigorous Vinyasa style of yoga places emphasis not just on yoga flows, but also on spiritual development and the interconnectedness of all beings. The five tenets of Jivamukti's philosophy are the study of scripture; devotion to God; meditation; learning to tune in to the vibrations of all matter; and nonharming (nonviolence) in mind, speech, and action. Along with flowing posture sequences, breathing, and meditation, some classes emphasize the importance of animal rights, veganism, and political activism.

Kundalini yoga
Through movement, chanting, breathing, and meditating, this type of yoga attempts to break through internal barriers and release energy to bring you to a higher level of self-awareness. Kundalini is a more spiritual practice emphasizing psychological and spiritual development along with physical health. Breathing exercises—some of them vigorous—are combined with a wide variety of posture and movement sequences. The practice is accessible to beginners and advanced practitioners alike.

Sivananda yoga
Sivananda yoga is another spiritual style focused on elevating the human consciousness. The practice consists of five elements: specific poses to enhance flexibility and improve circulation; deep, conscious breathing to reduce stress; relaxation to ease worry and fatigue; a vegetarian diet; and positive thinking. Classes tend to be slower-paced, and some include chanting.

Choosing a class
Once you have settled on a style (or styles) of yoga that would suit you, your next step is to find an actual class. Complicating the process, there are so many spin-offs from more traditional practices that it can be hard to tell the difference between them just by looking

at the name of the class. For example, hot yoga is similar to Bikram in that they're both done in a hot room, but the moves themselves are different. And there are hybrids such as Yogilates (a combination of yoga and Pilates) that don't give you a traditional practice of either one. Here are some clues to help you find a class that's appropriate for your level:

- If you go to a facility that offers only one type of yoga class, it's usually open to all levels. This means that the instructor should be offering modifications to make poses either easier or more challenging to accommodate all participants.
- Facilities that offer multiple classes may make it easier to choose by listing classes as level 1, 2, or 3 or by using descriptors like Extra Gentle Yoga, Gentle Yoga, Moderate Yoga, Challenging Yoga. Most yoga studios offer a wide variety of classes targeted to different populations.
- The facility you choose will often influence the type of yoga class you'll get. For example, a class at a senior center will likely be geared toward beginners, with more modifications for physical limitations. Classes at gyms and health clubs tend to lean more toward the physical fitness side of yoga. Specialty studios are likely to honor more traditional comprehensive practices.

After you've winnowed down the options, here are some questions you can ask to help ensure that the class you are considering is right for you.

What is the class like? Most facilities list class descriptions on their website. If you can't find enough detail, call. Describe your level of experience and ask which class would be best.

How quickly will you be moving from pose to pose? Generally, the faster the flow, the higher the intensity and level of challenge.

Are there tools to help modify poses? Straps, blocks, blankets, pillows, or pillow-like bolsters can help you to execute poses even if you're inflexible. Even if you've been practicing yoga for a while, when you try a new style, props may be helpful in the beginning. If a class offers them, it's a good sign that it accommodates multiple levels.

Who is the instructor? It's the instructor who really sets the tone of the class, so finding the right teacher is important (see "Finding a yoga teacher," below).

If you're unsure about a class, ask if you could simply observe it instead of participating your first time. Or skip it entirely. There are lots of yoga classes to choose from, and you want your first class to be a good experience.

Finding a yoga teacher

The National Center for Complementary and Integrative Health, a division of the National Institutes of Health, notes that yoga "is generally low-impact and safe for healthy people." But it immediately adds this qualifier—"when practiced appropriately under the guidance of a well-trained instructor." The following tips will help you find a good teacher.

Get references. Ask trusted sources to recommend a yoga teacher or studio. Some health practitioners are referring patients for yoga and may be good sources. Friends, family, and co-workers may be another source for recommendations, but ask people with levels of experience and fitness similar to yours in order to get the best recommendation for you. A yoga instructor who is right for your cousin who runs marathons may not be right for you if you're currently walking and have diabetes, for example.

Check qualifications. The Yoga Alliance, an independent nonprofit organization, maintains a registry of yoga instructors from various schools and yogic traditions who have received training that meets minimum standards in safety, anatomy, and yoga techniques and principles (see "Resources," page 53). Depending upon their training, instructors will be designated as a registered yoga teacher (RYT) or experienced registered yoga teacher (E-RYT). Both of these designations are usually followed by 200 or 500, indicating the number of hours of training the person received for credentials at that level. In addition, the Yoga

SPECIAL SECTION | Expand your practice—finding the right class

Alliance has designations for teachers trained in child yoga (RCYT) and prenatal yoga (RPYT). These are not certifications by the Yoga Alliance, but a verification that the instructor has completed approved training. Specific schools of yoga like Ashtanga, Bikram, Iyengar, or Kripalu have their own training requirements and programs.

Skip performers. These are instructors who stay at the front of the room the entire time, sometimes showing off what they can do. A high-quality instructor will be paying close attention to students and probably walking around and helping students make adjustments or modify poses to meet their individual needs.

Look for a welcoming environment. Instructors set the tone for the class. Look for one who is welcoming to all and makes you feel safe and comfortable, allowing you to proceed at your own pace. Competitive environments can encourage you to push yourself too far, risking an injury.

Ask about experience. This is key if you have any health or medical issues or limitations. Ideally, you should select an instructor who has experience working with your particular condition. If that's not possible, look for an instructor who will be attentive to your needs.

Avoiding injuries in class

No type of exercise—or any kind of activity, including climbing in and out of the bathtub—is 100% safe, so it's wise to be cautious. When you start taking classes, make sure that you're not pushing yourself beyond your limits. Following the guidelines listed here—in addition to the "Tips for a better, safer practice" on page 16—will help you avoid problems.

Talk to the instructor. Arrive early so you can introduce yourself to the teacher if you haven't already met. You should inform him or her that this is your first class or that you've never tried this particular style. Let the instructor know about your yoga experience, and mention any medical conditions or problems you have that may affect your ability. The teacher should be able to suggest ways you can modify poses—for example, using blocks to help support you in certain positions. He or she may also be able to show you alternate poses that are equally effective.

Do not attempt advanced classes if you're a beginner. At advanced levels, yoga can be quite difficult. You will be more likely to injure yourself if you jump right into advanced classes without building up through more basic levels first and developing needed skills as you go.

Realize that this is not a competition. If you're taking a class or watching a video, the instructor will be more flexible (not to mention more experienced) than you are. He or she will be able to stretch much farther than you likely can and enter more deeply into poses. Other members of the class may also be more advanced and more limber. Do not feel that you have to rival them. Instead, go only as far into a stretch or pose as your

Dangerous poses

Certain poses have been associated with serious risks, including nerve damage and strokes. Beginners and people with neck problems or circulatory issues should avoid the following poses:

- headstand
- shoulder stand
- plow
- wheel
- fish

body will comfortably allow. Over time, you'll become stronger and more flexible so you can do more safely. If you push yourself too far too fast, it can cause injuries.

Protect your neck. Avoid any pose that puts excessive pressure on your neck, such as the fish, plow, or shoulder stand poses, if you are a beginner or have any neck or circulatory issues. These poses may increase your risk for certain types of injuries, including nerve damage and even strokes (see "Dangerous poses," above).

Don't stress over yoga. Some research hints at a connection between mental strain and risk of injury. If yoga is feeling more stressful than positive, start more slowly, take it easier than usual, and bring more awareness to your practice. This will help to ease stress and protect you against injury.

Intermediate Yoga